"Transformation does not start with someone else changing you; transformation is an inner self reworking of what you are now to what you will be."

—Byron Pulsifer

"All the mindset work we talked about finally kicked in and it made a huge difference. Letting go of the negative self talk was instrumental. And all your principles of exercise and diet then worked once the mind shifted. Thank you. Down to 213 today (from 261)! 185 is in the sights now."

—Noah, 61, dentist

"I feel lighter and so much more energetic. I look leaner and a number of people have said that. Gaining muscle but losing fat. My cholesterol has improved too."

—Leon, 58, senior sales executive

"You are the best coaches. You really know how to tap in. As you mentioned before, change is emotional. I know I am strong, loved, valued, and worthy. I need to truly believe deep down."

—Nadine, 44, finance executive

"I have been battling this last year (hiding from family, except doctor) with my weight. I wanted you to know how inspiring you are to me and I'm sure with others no matter what they are struggling with in their life. My family was so proud and surprised of me this weekend for stepping out of my comfort zone. Thank you again for all you do . . . it does matter so much and inspires me to want to be 'the BEST ME!'"

—Tina, 58, sales executive

"Amazing journey guys! While I'm definitely looking forward to an occasional slice of bread or bowl of cereal, I absolutely see myself keeping up this lifestyle. The food choices were key. I didn't think I was doing too 'bad' before, but I wasn't doing too good either. Weight and A1C are both down! Thank you!"

—Larry, 50, IT executive

"Had my first 300-hour billable month since last year. Whenever I got crazy busy like this in the past, my weight would always go up. It was like a 1-to-1 correlation. But this time it's remained stable, which is really great!"

—Christopher, 41, attorney

"BTW . . . it's been two years since I completed your program and I still weigh within 1–3 lb from when I finished! I'm proud of that. I learned a lot about food and exercise that I continue to practice, so thank you!!!"

—Joan, 62, registered nurse

"I really was stuck for a long time and didn't know how to break through. I lost 40 lb using your method! My doctor is even on board with it. Thanks a lot, man!"

—Oscar, 48, venture capitalist

"It's really amazing; my metabolism has reset. When I'm good and follow your original plan, I lose weight. When I'm bad to the bone, I don't lose any weight, but I don't gain any weight, either . . . you guys jump-started my metabolism!"

—Jill, 55, IT executive

the nine shifts

THE MIND-FIRST METHOD TO TRANSFORM YOUR BODY AND YOUR LIFE

DEEKRON KRIKORIAN, MBA

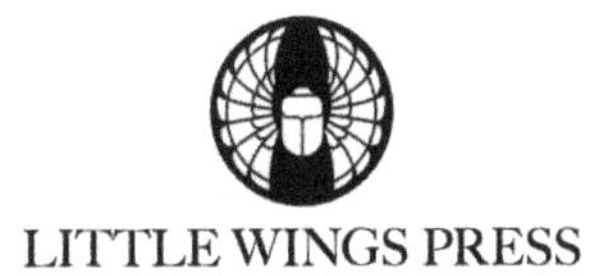

LITTLE WINGS PRESS

Published in the United States by Little Wings Press
www.littlewingspress.com

ISBN 979-8-9893149-0-4 (Hardcover Edition)
ISBN 979-8-9893149-1-1 (Paperback Edition)
ISBN 979-8-9893149-2-8 (eBook Edition)

First Edition: January 2024

Book Design & Cover by Adam "Adameus" Levine
Illustrated by Megan Douglas

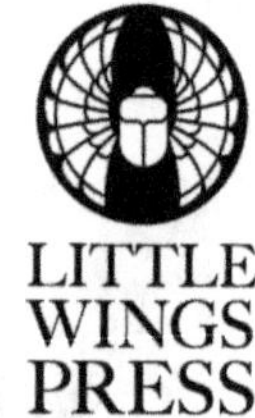

LITTLE
WINGS
PRESS

For Ma and Ta.
Thank you for making me.
(And for making me who I am.)
Mulțumesc
Շնորհակալութիւն

Contents

PART III: THE SOLUTION

PART IV: YOUR FUTURE

Case Studies

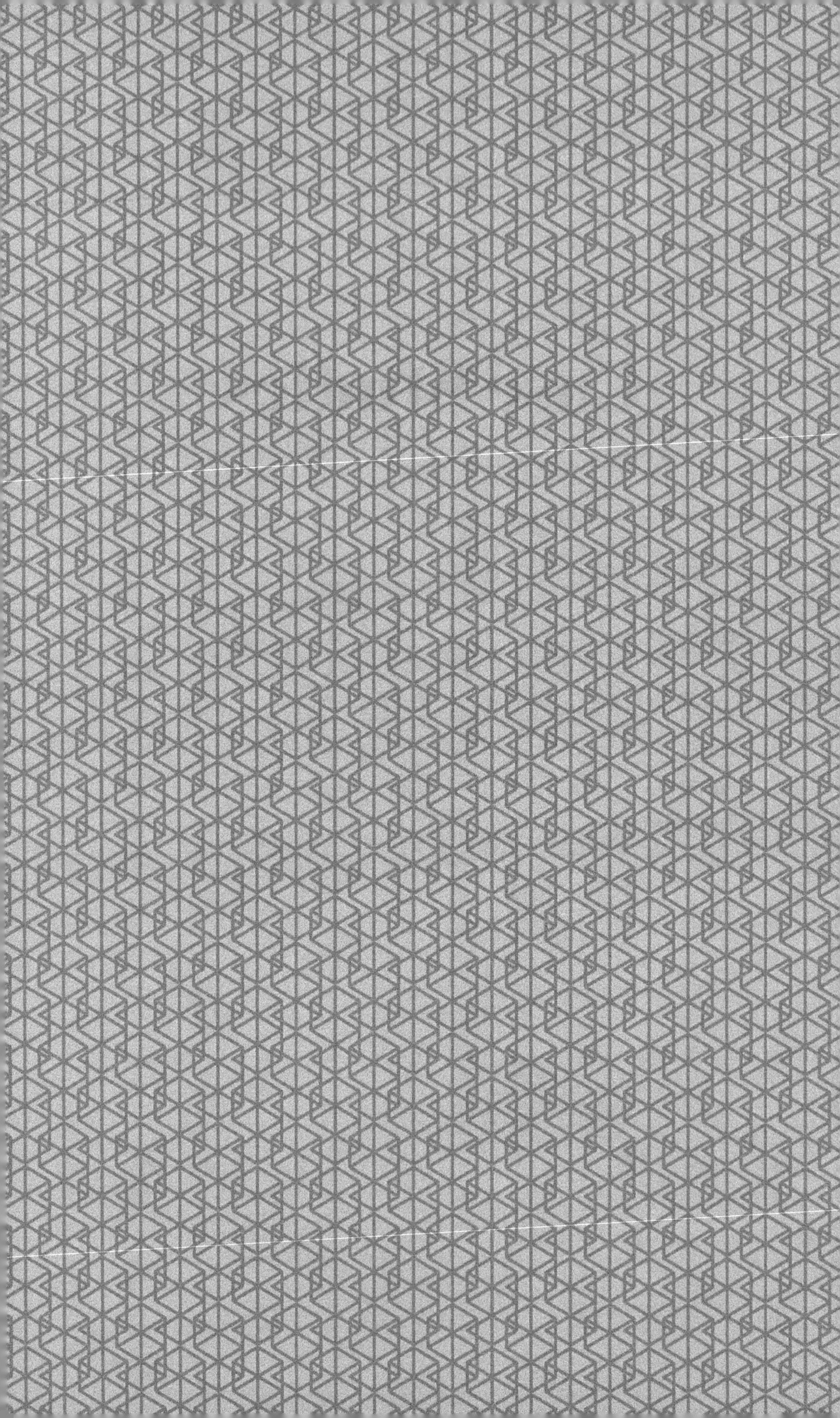

the nine shifts

THE MIND-FIRST METHOD
TO TRANSFORM YOUR BODY
AND YOUR LIFE

Introduction

"Your ultimate goal in life is to become your best self. Your immediate goal is to get on the path that will lead you there."
—David Viscott

You and I have something in common. As beings who walk this earth during a short stint of human experience, we want to make the most of our time here. And unless the ancient Egyptians were right, there is no afterlife. This means you and I only get one shot to live our best possible life in the years we have available. If that's true, then we have to consistently bring the best version of ourself, every day.

Obviously, this is easier said than done.

Our thought patterns, Father Time, and life's challenges can all get in the way of us living the kind of life we seek.

Overcoming what's in our way requires both a desire to be better and the knowledge for how to get there.

Having the right guide or mentor also helps (a lot).

I've been that guide for many people.

Leading folks to achieve the best versions of themself is something I'm highly passionate about.

That's because I've had the good fortune to have had some great guides. The transformations I've achieved—in both my mind and my body—have made all the difference in empowering me to live my best life.

And I want the same for you.

THIS BOOK WILL INSPIRE YOU TO CHANGE AND SHOW YOU HOW TO GET THERE

For starters, you have this book and are about to see how to implement my proven transformation method, *The Nine Shifts.*

Congrats to you for picking it up. It tells me that the desire is in your heart to reach higher and create a better future.

If so, know that *The Nine Shifts* will guide you to achieve the very best version of you.

It's a collection of wisdom that I've gained over a 20+ year personal development journey, a 30+ year body transformation journey, years spent as a former strategy consultant creating frameworks, and a 5+ year journey of intimately coaching over 120 professionals one-on-one in achieving a lasting transformation in mind and body.

I wrote it to inspire you to change by sharing some of my clients' success stories. Hearing about how they overcame their struggles, some of which you, yourself may be facing, will re-energize you and show you that long-lasting change in your body is possible to achieve—even if it has eluded you for a long time.

I also wrote it to show you how to change, and do it in way that's:

- **Doable**—by making manageable shifts.
- **Clear**—by following a straightforward framework that eliminates confusion.
- **Appropriate**—by accounting for potential complications due to age, hormones, or past injuries.
- **Comprehensive**—by addressing how life's obligations and distractions can get in the way of our habits.
- **Permanent**—by working deeply at the level of your mind and emotions to shift your behavior for good.

You can think of it as a playbook for what I call "Mind-First Transformation." That's when we go on a journey to permanently elevate our mind, body, and life (versus when we watch some content about mindset but forget about it, lose a few pounds by going on a diet but gain it back, or making small changes in our habits that don't last very long).

GET READY TO LOOK, FEEL, AND PERFORM YOUR BEST

The framework in this book focuses on creating lasting change in your body and health, because as they say, health is the ultimate wealth. Without our health (or a high-functioning body), it's impossible to live our best life.

If you're struggling with your body because you are carrying excess weight, feeling low in energy, or are concerned about your future because your health markers are elevated, this book will help you get out of this "debt" so you can feel healthy and in control again.

If you're doing OK in your body, this book will give you the tools to become optimal. To go beyond "normal" or average, to experiencing superior energy, function, and longevity. Not to mention, to look great and exude maximum confidence.

Ultimately, it's your bible on how to look, feel, and perform your best.

It was written with over-40 professionals in mind but the science-based principles will work for anyone, regardless of age or career.

HOW TO READ THIS BOOK

The first few chapters of the book will set the stage for your transformation by showing you what's possible on the other side (and that it actually is possible to get there). Then, I will go over what I've identified as the nine primary challenges standing in the way of us achieving lasting change in our body and health. They are grouped into the categories of Mind, Body, and Life. Three categories with three challenges under each.

After you get a sense of which of the challenges have been tripping you up and why, you'll learn how to overcome each of those nine challenges by making nine shifts in the areas of your Mindset, Metabolism, and Momentum. To guide you in making each shift, you will find an action plan in each of the shift chapters.

The action plans include everything from mindset transformation exercises, an example meal plan, workout routines, sleep hygiene practices, to strategies for when you travel, and more. I recommend you do the exercises (and download the free resources) for each of the shift chapters, especially the ones that address a challenge with which you may be struggling now.

While the book covers some complex topics in the areas of both psychology (e.g., motivation, limiting beliefs) and physiology (e.g., metabolism, nutrition) I racked my brain to keep them as simple and as user-friendly as possible for you.

I suggest you read the book in its entirety to understand how all the pieces fit. Then, review the chapters for the challenges with which you've struggled—and their corresponding shift chapters—so you can learn how to overcome those challenges.

NOT EASY BUT WORTH IT (AND WE CAN SUPPORT YOU IN GETTING THERE)

Real transformation work is not easy but it's well worth it because it elevates your entire life in a lasting way. Just know that it takes patience, a commitment to continuous progress, and being "bigger" than your obstacles.

If you get stuck, or want to speed up the process (while ensuring you implement things the right way), know that my team and I are here to support your journey.

We've gotten really good at empowering clients to overcome their challenges and work through their complications, including mental obstacles, hormonal imbalances (like high blood sugar, low testosterone, menopause, etc.), and insane schedules.

When you're ready, know that you can connect for a quick, complimentary intro call with us anytime at the following link: https://thenineshifts.com/call

For the rest of you, I salute you for taking a bold step to learn, grow, and transform.

I trust the journey you're about to take with the help of this book will be valuable, life-changing, and body-changing.

I'm waiting for you on the other side.

Here's to being our best.

Yours in greatness,

Dikran "Deekron" Krikorian

Chief Transformation Officer at The InPowerment Company™

PART I

The Situation

CHAPTER 1

Why We Struggle

"I can't remember the last time I looked in the mirror and liked what I saw."

Tracy couldn't even look at me, her voice just above a whisper. "I'm so ashamed."

Near tears, she let it all out. "Not just in the boardroom, Deekron. In the bedroom, too. I'm constantly embarrassed. I never look at my reflection if I can help it."

Her confidence was shattered.

As hard as it was, I knew at that moment what Tracy needed was for me to listen to her. To hear her and see her. So I listened. I heard. I saw.

"There's more," she said.

"Tell me."

"My A1C has gone up," she said, "I'm officially prediabetic."

She paused.

"I'm scared, Deekron. I'm forty-five and I'm afraid if I don't find a way to somehow change what's happening to me, I'm going to end up . . . I'm afraid I'm going to be a total failure."

She had censored herself there, but we both knew what she really meant. She was frightened that she'd become a disappointment to herself and her family. Terrified that she may become dangerously unhealthy as she aged, and all the scary words that come with that, like cancer, heart attack, and stroke. She knew that one day she was going to retire from being a corporate attorney for a tech giant, and she wanted to have enough health left to enjoy it. She had tried, over and over again, with various health programs and schemes. But she wasn't able to maintain her progress for very long, and now the state of her body and her health was consuming her.

Tracy continued, "I've tried. I've tried so many times. I've tried eating healthier. I've tried running. I've tried quitting wine. Nothing works. And now I'm not sure if anything will work. I have no idea what I'm doing. I have no idea if I'm doing it right. I'm constantly thinking about whether I can or can't eat something, or how I'll fit in exercise, or when I'm going to exercise, or whether I can stay in bed for another hour or have to get up and go for a run, or whether I even need to go for a run."

I kept listening, my heart breaking for her.

I knew exactly how Tracy was feeling.

She wasn't prepared to accept a fate where she is not in control of her body and her health.

She was frantic to turn things around and not feel ashamed about her body anymore.

I could relate to her struggle. It took me decades to finally get my body to where I wanted it to be. During my own battle, I'd feel frustrated and defeated, more times than I'd like to admit.

No matter how much I'd obsess over getting my body to change, after a short spell of progress, something would happen and I'd be knocked off track. Making progress, only to regress and find myself back at square one was a very familiar and disheartening experience.

I later found out that I wasn't alone.

LOTS OF US ARE STRUGGLING

Turns out that most people today, especially in the U.S., are struggling with their body and their health. Consider some of these statistics:

- Over 73% of the U.S. population is overweight, over 42% are obese, and the numbers keep growing.[1]

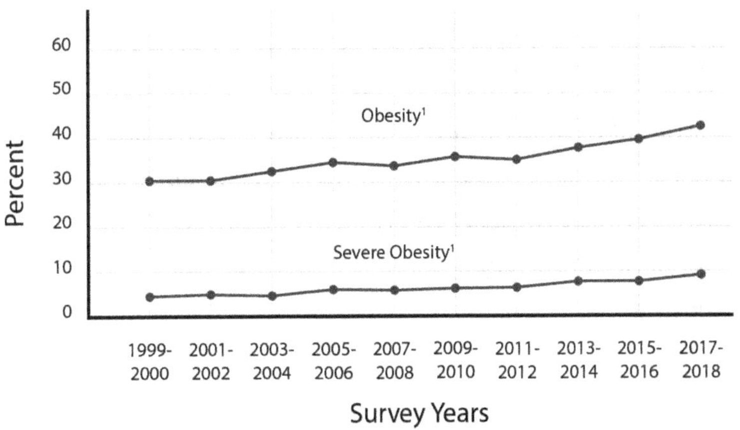

- Only 12% of Americans are considered "metabolically healthy."[2]
- The average American gains close to 50 lb between the ages of twenty and sixty due to metabolic decline, hormonal changes, and lifestyle factors.[3]
- Weight related diseases are on the rise. In 1958, around one million Americans had Type 2 diabetes. By 2018, the number had grown to 34 million.[4]
- Gaining just 10–20 lb begins to increase the risk of death. Becoming obese accelerates premature death by 50–100%.[5]

To say that those statistics are alarming doesn't quite cover it. It was no surprise to me that Tracy was scared out of her mind thinking about her possible future. The consequences of staying in a mentally and physically unfit state are terrifying. Not just for Tracy, or for me; for all of us.

We've all seen this in our families and our communities. We lose some of them too young, or we lose them in a different way as they become a shadow of their formerly vibrant, healthy selves. None of us wants to be the one who creates a burden on our children or loved ones by relying on them to care for us doing basic things that were once in our control. And, of course, none of us wants to experience the pain and suffering that comes with things like diabetes, high blood pressure, cancer or heart disease.

What should be obvious after reading Tracy's story, and all of the statistics above, is that being unfit and unhealthy is a huge risk to our self-image, quality of life, and longevity.

The stakes are too high for us, and those around us, to get this wrong.

THE DECK IS NOT IN YOUR FAVOR

On top of all of that, the cards are stacked against us. Here's what I mean.

OUR ENVIRONMENT CONDITIONS US TO MAKE UNHEALTHY FOOD CHOICES

In 2023, more than 200,000 fast food restaurants were operating in the U.S. Over 80% of families eat fast food at least once per week, while a third of us are eating it every day.[6] A full 73% of the foods in the U.S. food supply fit the definition of "ultra-processed."[7] These convenient, low-cost, chemically processed foods are engineered to hit the reward centers in our brain and trigger dopamine by being tasty, satisfying, and high in calories. They're also directly correlated to health issues such as obesity, diabetes, and cardiovascular disease, all while being slickly packaged and heavily marketed. Collectively, the food industry is the second largest advertiser in the U.S., only after retail.[8] We're constantly being conditioned to consume cheap, convenient, and addicting foods, to the long-term detriment of our health. With an overabundance of low-quality, highly-processed foods within arms reach, it's no wonder we're becoming more and more unhealthy.

WE'RE DROWNING IN (MIS)INFORMATION

These days, thanks to the internet and social media, there's a tsunami of advice about how to lose weight, get in shape, change your diet, and more. As of this writing, Instagram has:

- twenty-seven million posts tagged #keto
- seventy-seven million posts tagged #diet
- eighty-eight million posts tagged #weightloss
- five-hundred million (yes, over half a billion!) posts tagged #fitness.

The deluge of information ranges from the over-simplified (calories in, calories out) to the wildly complex (scientific studies, far-out biohacks). Some of it can be helpful, but it's too hard to piece together in a way that's relevant. Most of it is not helpful. It can either be conflicting (at best), or deceptive (at worst); selling us some product that probably won't work and we likely don't need.

KEEPING OUR BODY IN A GREAT PLACE CONSISTENTLY IS HARD

Studies show that 90% of dieters regain any weight they lost during a diet, and 92% of New Year's weight-loss resolutions go unmet.[9] There's many reasons for this, including setting unrealistic goals and relying on willpower to power through unsustainable approaches like restrictive diets or extreme workouts. Suffice it to say that if you've failed to achieve lasting success in keeping your health and fitness where you want it, you're not alone.

HOW WE GET IN OUR OWN WAY

Another source of our struggles is actually ourselves—our mind, our body, and our life all get in the way of keeping our body where we want it. As you will soon see, there are many reasons why the mind, with its survival-based tendencies, will resist change and sabotage our habits.

Next is the body with its metabolism, hormones, and other physiological systems that are constantly adapting. Oftentimes we cause the wrong adaptations that can lead to excess body fat, low energy, or poor health without us even realizing it. Not to mention the natural changes and decline that take place in the body as we age.

Finally, our life trips us up by getting in the way of our habits by throwing commitments and curveballs our way.

Most people don't have a strategy to deal with these obstacles and struggle with a body they don't want as a result.

MOST PRODUCTS AND SERVICES DON'T WORK VERY WELL (OR FOR VERY LONG)

If we turn to products and services to help with this challenge, they usually leave us disappointed. They either don't work very well, or if they do, they don't work for very long. There are a number of reasons for this, which I will be getting into. Here's a quick summary.

The majority of products that are "weight loss" or metabolism focused, like supplements, do very little to drive meaningful change in the body. (Nope, there's no "magic pill.")

In addition, many approaches and services are temporary in nature. First, because they focus too much on cutting calories, dieting, or restriction (e.g., counting calories, or Keto). This makes them too hard to sustain; plus, they slow your metabolism in the process. Second, because they are purposely time-bound (e.g., a 21-day Fat Loss Challenge, 6-week bootcamp), when they end, you're back to square one. Third, because they mostly focus on the basics of meals or workouts paired with some basic accountability (e.g., personal trainers, typical online fitness coaches). Most of these folks, though well meaning, lack the skill to create long-term behavior change by addressing your ingrained beliefs, thought patterns, emotions, habits, and life obstacles. You may succeed while on the program, but once you're off, your old habits—and your old shape—can come right back.

This keeps most people on what I call the "weight loss hamster wheel," constantly losing weight, regressing, and searching for the next thing that will help them lose the weight again.

So yeah, our environment, ourselves, and the solutions we turn to are all working against us.

Wow.

Is it any wonder why people, especially in the U.S., struggle to have the long-term success with their body or their health that they want? Yes, some people do succeed. But, most do not. Those that do succeed, especially without the right strategy and support, are the exception. Trying to solve this puzzle amidst a lack of knowledge, high stress, and limited time—the norm for most over-40 professionals—can seem harder than running a marathon in the rain, blindfolded, with your feet tied together.

Not easy.

It certainly wasn't easy for me. I struggled, too. For a really long time.

Thirty years, in fact.

It was hard for Tracy, and I know it's hard for many of us.

For the majority of us, it's a constant game of trying something for a little while (e.g., a diet, workout plan, or supplement), making some progress, but then falling off track and regressing in our body. Consistency can be an elusive son of a gun.

Regrettably, failing at this can leave us feeling terrible and inept. And it can feel daunting—even hopeless—to keep trying. Especially after so many past failed attempts. I mean, how much frustration are we supposed to endure?

CHAPTER 2

A Better Way

"The true sense of intelligence is not
knowledge but imagination."
—Albert Einstein

What if keeping your body and health where you want them didn't have to be a frustrating, start-again, stop-again process that leaves us feeling stuck, unhealthy, ashamed, or powerless? What if there's a different future available for you, for us, that is so much better than the one painted in all of those scary statistics? A future where you are confident in your abilities to be in control of your body and health. One where you look, feel and perform your best, year-round, into your golden age?

Can you imagine it?

I'm here to say that it's completely possible (if you really *want* it and it is important to you).

In Shakespeare's play The Tragedy of Julius Caesar, Roman general Mark Antony famously pleads, "Friends, Romans, countrymen, lend me your ears!"

My turn.

"High achievers, ambitious types, and go-getters, lend me your imagination!"

WHAT IF LIFE COULD BE LIKE THIS?

Picture it:

- You wake up in the morning well rested and inspired.
- Your simple but strategic morning ritual empowers your mind and body. Your blood is flowing, your metabolism is in high gear. You're connected with your heart, focused in your mind, and clear about your day ahead.
- You're intentional about your most important priorities. You're at peace, knowing you're in control, regardless of what comes your way. You're ready to handle any stress or curveball that people or life may throw at you.
- You feel great about how your clothes fit you and have the freedom to wear anything in your closet, including your favorite pair of jeans or that skinny black dress you bought decades ago.
- You start work, brimming with confidence at meetings, presentations, and Zoom calls.
- You're full of energy and clarity. You interact with your team effectively and with certainty.
- You know how to fit your important habits in, even on days full of back-to-back meetings or when you're on the road.
- You eat meals and hydrate smartly to support your

best mental and physical functioning. You know what nutrition is best for you, and how different foods affect your body.

- You know which workouts are optimal for you, and you do them regularly to stay strong, lean, and fit. They keep you mobile, functional, and free from aches or pains.
- You make it through the end of each day feeling productive and proud.
- Your newfound productivity and mental clarity allow you to produce more but work less.
- Even after a long day, you have energy left over to give to the people and hobbies you love when you get home.
- You feel good when you're in social situations, confident in your own skin and ready to smile for the camera or take a selfie.
- You have the luxury of enjoying good food and drink when you're out for an occasion. You're comfortable knowing those special events won't impact your health or waistline, and you don't obsess over every little thing you put in your mouth.
- You're in peak health, and thoughts of scary conditions like diabetes, cancer, heart disease, or stroke rarely, if ever, cross your mind.

Basically, you feel pretty unstoppable.

In this future—the one with this unstoppable version of you—you're in a groove with a strategic set of mind and body transformation habits that you mastered from what you learned in this book. These habits are part of your ongoing lifestyle. You fit them in easily without much time or thought. They ensure you stay optimal by keeping your mind calm and resilient, your metabolism and energy high, your body lean and fit, your health primed and your life firing on all cylinders. Your mental health, health habits, and lifestyle are on autopilot.

You've learned how to make shifts in your mind, your body, and your life so you can be and bring your best, every day.

Does it seem impossible to actually live this way?

From where you're standing right now, it may indeed feel unattainable.

It's not.

(And I wrote this book to prove it.)

DOES IT SEEM OUT OF REACH?

Right now, you might be skeptical. I'm telling you this "fairy tale story" about how life can be, and you're ready to throw the book across the room. You're probably thinking, "Deekron! What the heck are you talking about? I've tried! I've tried ALL THE THINGS. Dammit, man, you're talking nonsense!"

Yup. I get it.

If you've tried and failed many times to bring your body to a good place then the life I just described may seem like it's out of reach.

Stay with me. I promise it'll make sense.

I remember how frustrated I was during the decades that I kept struggling to hold on to my body transformation progress. I went through many cycles of starting and stopping. Making progress for a while, but then regressing whenever life would throw me a curveball or my motivation would wane. I felt like a loser.

Similarly, many of my clients, even the highest achievers, come to me with their confidence at an all-time low, concerned about their health and limited in their abilities. They long for more confidence, higher energy levels, greater conviction in themselves, more peace of mind around their future, and fewer aches and pains. More than that, they don't want their physical state to limit their success or create a burden on those around them.

I get it.

But take heart because there is indeed a better way to achieve the future you've been craving.

It just might not be what you're expecting.

I'm not here to reveal some new weight loss hack, fitness fad, quick-fix supplement or fancy injection.

I'm here to show you what I truly believe is something better.

A BETTER WAY

Attaining and maintaining your body and health in an optimal place over time comes down to one main thing.

Make this one change in your approach and you'll never get set back or regress.

Once I made it, I hit my goals, reached my peak physical shape, and never relapsed again.

You know that amazing life and future I described above? This one change has helped me enjoy all those amazing benefits—peak health, performance, energy, confidence—year-round.

The one change in your approach you have to make is simply this (drum roll, please):

Instead of just focusing on how to change your body, start by first focusing on your mind.

Instead of directing your efforts towards only diet and exercise, take an "inside-out approach" and begin your body transformation journey with the mind.

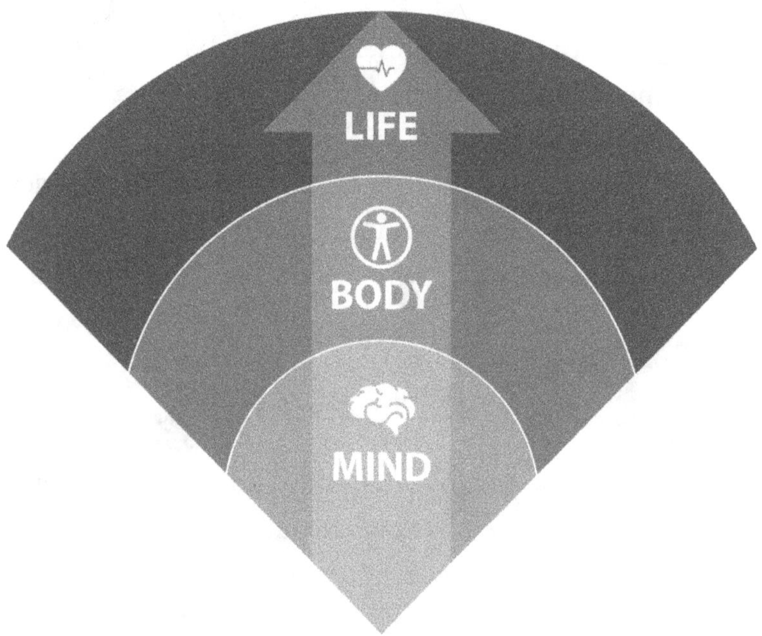

Without first changing the mind, our progress is sure to be short-lived, at best.

I mean, think about it. The mind and the body are connected, aren't they?

So, why would we try to change one without changing the other?

Yet, this is what almost everyone does.

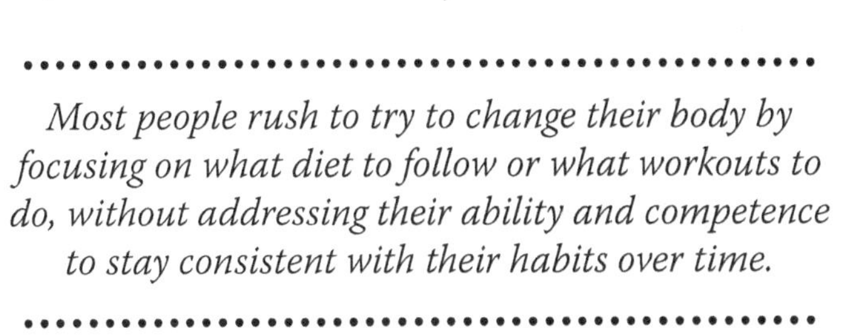

Most people rush to try to change their body by focusing on what diet to follow or what workouts to do, without addressing their ability and competence to stay consistent with their habits over time.

Tony Robbins says that success is only 20% strategy and 80% psychology.

Unfortunately, the large majority of folks are focused on finding the perfect strategy. They seek out the latest diet, supplement, or workout class. They follow generic advice from random online sources or influencers. They may follow it for a little while, but what do they do when obstacles come up, like when procrastination kicks in? Or when they get overwhelmed by work or life demands? When their motivation is down? When they're not seeing progress and feel like quitting? When they're feeling like they're destined to be overweight? When cravings get the best of them?

It's these mind-related obstacles we have to get good at managing if we want to be successful over the long run.

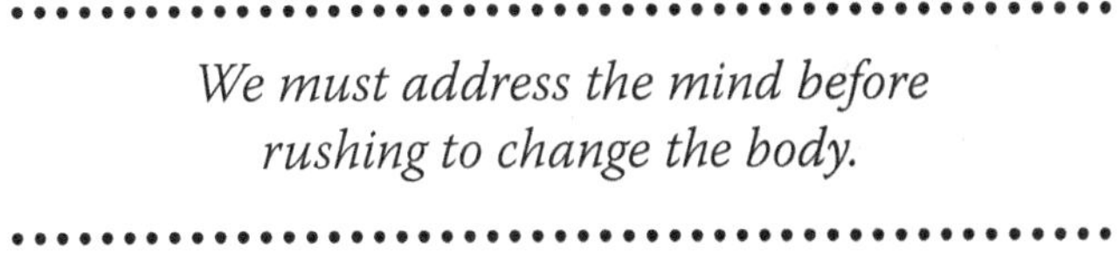

We must address the mind before rushing to change the body.

Then, and only then, we work on changing the body—by using the ***right*** strategies. This is especially important if we're over-40. Strategies that focus on boosting an aging metabolism instead of cutting calories (which slows your metabolism). Strategies like using age-appropriate workouts designed to your available time and abilities. Strategies that have you prepared to prevent all of life's interruptions from throwing you off your game.

If you're starting to get the sense that it's essential to address *all* of the pieces of the puzzle—mind, body, and life—not just diet and exercise alone, then you're already on your way!

It wasn't until I addressed all the pieces together that I was able to achieve lasting results and keep them, day after day, week after week, and year after year. Only by using a mind-first, comprehensive approach can we see long term change, transforming and maintaining our minds, bodies, and lives where we want them to be, over the long run.

This "inside-out" approach may be new to you but it's what's required for you to finally succeed.

HOW I FINALLY TRANSFORMED MY BODY FOR GOOD

Human beings are slow to change.

Jennifer Kunst, PhD writes in Psychology Today, "There is an enormous pressure in the human psyche to maintain the status quo."[10] Sometimes we don't make a change until we feel like our back is against the wall.

That was certainly the case with me.

In 2015, when I was in my mid-forties, the tech startup that I had co-founded, Motion Traxx, was in trouble. User acquisition was slowing, well-funded copycat competitors had entered the space, and we were running out of money, fast. My company was facing bankruptcy and I was dealing with the disappointment and frustration that came from my beloved company falling apart.

If that wasn't bad enough, I was also going through a divorce.

Everything fell apart, all at once. (When it rains, it pours!)

I had to move out of my home, find a new source of income, and basically start my entire life over again (as a middle-aged, divorced guy, no less).

I was so stressed and anxious about my future that worrying about my health habits or achieving my dream body was the last thing on my mind. It felt like a luxury I couldn't afford.

But I kept feeling this nudge from inside.

"Deekron," it said, "you can't afford ***not*** to be your best right now."

Like most people, I ignored it. But it kept at me.

"Deekron," it said, "finally getting in great shape and peak health is the best possible thing you could do for your life right now."

"Oh, please," I said. "I don't have time for that!"

"DAMMIT DEEKRON," it said, "YOU'VE BEEN WANTING THIS FOR SO LONG!!!"

(It was true. I had been pretty obsessed with putting on muscle and looking my best as a man since the young age of 13 when I started lifting weights in my dad's basement.)

That's when I realized the truth—the truth that, in the midst of my despair, I was not seeing.

Improving my body was exactly what I needed to turn my life around.

Having a healthy body would give me more confidence, more mental clarity, and more energy. Those things would give me what I desperately needed to tackle and succeed in all of the areas of my life that were failing—career, health, and relationships. My body was the motor that would drive success in all areas of my life. It was so clear to me. Despite being overwhelmed, divorced, and anxious about the path my life would take, I vowed to be the healthiest, fittest version of myself that I was capable of.

When I finally doubled-down on achieving this goal, I dove in (hard). I spent countless hours reading books about nutrition and metabolism, watching videos about exercise science on YouTube, tracking and analyzing my food and training data, working with elite coaches, and even rubbing elbows with hardcore bodybuilders. I immersed myself in this world, learning—and trying—everything I could find. Some of it worked and some of it didn't, but I got really smart about the science of changing the body.

Yet, even with all of that trying, the results were erratic; one step forward and two steps back. It was hard to keep regular consistency with these new habits I was learning. At first I blamed my situation—my mind's default cop out. But one morning as I woke up, it hit me like a ton of bricks: I needed to shift my thinking. I had to put my mind first to overcome obstacles that were getting in the way. Instantly, I was transported back to the personal development work I had done about a decade earlier, when I was in my mid-thirties.

At that time, I had also hit a wall. I was feeling stuck in my career, dealing with anxiety, having heart palpitations, and feeling unfulfilled. My first cousin, trying very hard to help me, invited me to come check out a transformation program she had been doing, and loving. Initially, I thought it was a bunch of rah-rah baloney and said "thanks but no thanks." I'd figure it out, I was sure. But I didn't. The stuckness and lack of fulfillment went on, and on, ***and on***. Eventually I got to my breaking point. I'd had enough. I was ready to try anything.

So I called up my cousin, a little sheepishly, and asked if that invite was still open. Fortunately for me it was and I signed up for that program. ***BAM!*** At the risk of sounding like an infomercial, I must say: it truly and completely changed my life. The powerful mindset transformation and the greater self-awareness I gained helped me be way more at peace and a lot more grounded—to be more fulfilled and more connected to my real self and those around me. They gave me the courage to speak up and take risks in a way I couldn't before, including boldly leaving a prestigious career in corporate America as a strategy consultant to pursue my passion of helping people with their health.

That memory galvanized me, and I knew I needed to start using all of those mental and emotional transformation skills again. ***BAM!*** I started to heal and elevate my mind in the aftermath of the divorce, and then I took those same skills and applied them to my whole self—rewiring my mind along with my body and my life.

I started to have breakthroughs, one after the other.

With each one, somehow, almost like magic, my ability to keep the body habits that were propelling me forward got easier and easier.

Being more clear, more grounded, and less reactionary to what life would throw at me helped me to be more consistent with my habits and more unstoppable in the face of obstacles.

Understanding how I was wired and uncovering blindspots about myself and my thought patterns helped me to listen less to old fears and be easier on myself, even when I failed at things (like not seeing results in my body or my business). I had more freedom and more time because I was freed from the old me who was constantly trying so hard to prove himself and be perfect all the time.

Combining those mental and emotional tools with what I had already learned about health and fitness completely changed everything about the way I approached my mind, my body, and my life.

Through trial and error, I boiled everything down to a science-based set of components that gave me what I needed to be my healthiest and fittest, both mentally and physically. Then, I strapped on my strategy consultant hat and assembled all of those components into a strategic system that was efficient and sustainable enough to work for me as a busy professional over-40 in the midst of major life changes.

Over time, I refined and improved this system I had created. I made it easier, more efficient, more seamless. As I tweaked and integrated this system, I was able to maintain my habits regularly and effortlessly. My body completely transformed—thanks to the transformation that I had done on my mind—and everything changed for the better.

Today, I look, feel, and perform my best, year-round, and I sustain it with a set of effective and efficient habits that take just 3–5 hours per week.

I carry myself with confidence in all situations, work, social, or otherwise.

I spend more time growing my two health & wellness businesses and helping people. I spend more time with friends and family. I spend more time traveling (for fun) and never worry when I miss my workouts for a few days while on the road. I have so many things that I am grateful for today:

- Muscle and strength, plus mobility. I never think twice about running up a flight of stairs to catch a train, picking up a heavy box off the ground, or going for a 5k run with a friend.
- More confidence in business and in social situations, including dating.
- More energy that is sustained throughout the day and into the evening. No 3 pm crashes or food comas.
- Clarity around my key habits each day and week, so I always know what needs to get done.
- Mental energy that keeps me grounded, inspired, and driving forward in all areas.
- Freedom to enjoy travel or holidays without worrying about any backsliding.
- Power to tackle tough deadlines or hard work without losing track of my key habits.

My life is like this now because of the smart and strategic body transformation system I created, which I call *The Nine Shifts.*

Want to know the best part?

I have a lot of wiggle room to eat and drink as it suits my plans. Having something sinful makes little difference to my waistline, and feeling guilty about what I just consumed is a thing of the past. In fact, at the ripe age of fifty-two, I maintain a lean, strong body (complete with six-pack abs) all year round. (I live in Miami. It's in the rules.) I'm proud to say that I usually have one of the better bodies when I'm at the beach or the pool.

You may not care too much about some of these things, like looking good at the pool. That's okay. I know that I'm a bit crazy (and kinda vain) in my own way. We all have different priorities, which is why every person's motives for going on a transformation journey are going to look a little bit different.

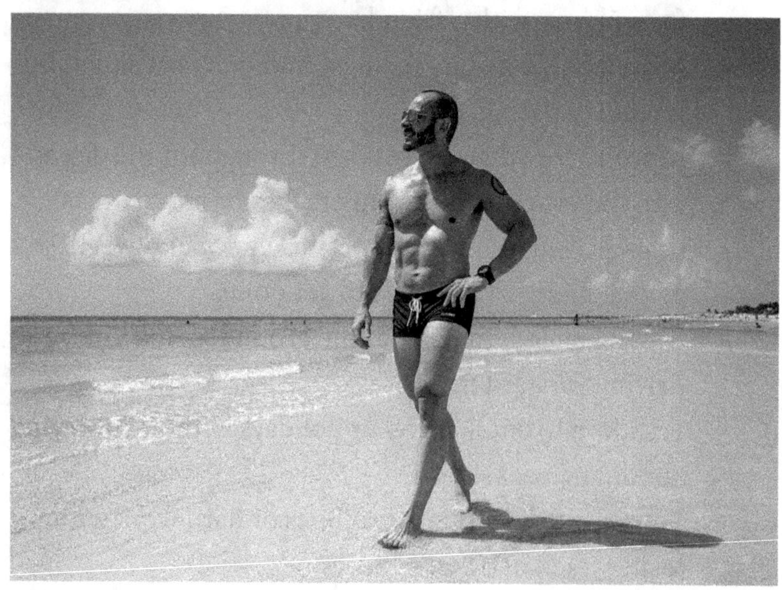

Suffice it to say that transforming my mind and body has made all the difference in turning my life around and being able to consistently be the best version of myself.

So, that's (the short version) of my story.

Now, let me share a few of my client success stories, so you can see how each of us chooses to transform in a slightly different way, while having to overcome different challenges and circumstances.

SOME OF MY FAVORITE CLIENT SUCCESS STORIES

This approach doesn't only work for me. I've seen it over and over again: when I coach my clients to work on their mind first—rewiring their thought patterns to manage negative emotions, changing limiting beliefs, and tapping into true motivation—they gain the tools to sustain their results for a lifetime. This is why I do deep work with my clients and why, in this book, we're going to talk about transforming your mind as the first step to transforming your body.

Below are some of my favorite client success stories (you'll find some more sprinkled throughout the book). Their names have been changed to protect their privacy, but everything I have to say about them (and they say about themselves) is absolutely true.

Their journey toward personal growth, and their newfound health and confidence, are very inspiring to me. I trust that they will inspire you, too.

- **Tammy, a 57-year-old finance executive.** Thin for most of her life, going through menopause and caring for an aging mom caused Tammy to gain seventy pounds and develop prediabetes. She felt heavy and hated how she looked in photos. She felt like a deer in the headlights, she was struggling to find the motivation to take that first step, and was even confused about what the right first step should be given her age and situation (she never had to lose weight before). After working with me on *The Nine Shifts* Tammy was able to lose close to 30 lb, reduce her menopause belly significantly, and feel lighter in her body with a lot more energy.

- **Deborah, a 52-year-old owner of a leading real estate agency.** A former IronMan triathlete whose busy schedule made it hard to stick to a routine, Deborah had added unwanted pounds and was feeling bad about her body and herself. It certainly didn't help that she, unfortunately, wasn't getting much support from those around her at home. This made her feel like not even bothering. She reached out for us to be the lifeline she needed. Today, she has a flexible system that works with her busy schedule, and allows her to stay at her target weight. She says, "*The Nine Shifts* cuts through all the muck and BS out there. This is not a diet."
- **Stacy, a 60-year-old senior software sales executive.** Heavy travel, having to meet sales quotas, and managing her sales team led to falling off balance and neglecting her health for years. "I've let my job get the best of me," she bemoaned. This left her feeling terrible about her body, health, and future. Stacy also dealt

with Hashimoto's Syndrome, a disorder that leads to an underactive thyroid and makes it hard to lose weight. With our support and specific recommendations around metabolism habits and lifestyle, she has a plan that works with her busy schedule. "I got solid guidance on how you lose weight and increase your metabolism. It's been life changing!" she celebrated.

- **Walter, a 47-year old program manager and former decorated officer.** A severe injury knocked Walter off of his health routine. Stress eating and low testosterone caused an extra fifty pounds to come on. This shattered his confidence and led to major guilt, making him feel like he was being a bad father. Today, he fits way better in his clothes and, thanks to his newfound confidence from getting his prior, fit body back, Walter was able to get a more fulfilling and higher paying job.
- **Nancy, a 64-year-old legal assistant.** Stress from caring for her aging parents led Nancy to stress eat, causing weight gain and blood sugar levels elevating into the pre-diabetic range. She was appalled; never did she think she was going to end up like her parents, both of whom were Type 2 diabetics living in long-term care. Today, thanks to the blood sugar management techniques and fat loss reduction habits we helped her adopt, she has reduced her A1C from a pre-diabetic to a healthy level and is ecstatic about it. She wrote us saying "I did it! My A1C went from 6.2 to 5.6. I'm ecstatic. This was huge for me, Deekron."

- **Jill, a 55-year-old IT executive.** Jill works from home and sits all day long. This, and going through menopause, caused her to gain unwanted body fat, primarily in her love handles. She was frustrated by this and even more by the fact that all the things she had been trying, like walking and online fitness classes, weren't working. Today, she has a routine and lifestyle that lets her work from home and keep off the extra body fat.
- **Eric, a 65-year-old former airline industry executive.** After his partner was struck and killed by a car, Eric was devastated. He needed time to fully process his grief. When he emerged from his healing, he wanted to feel confident and healthy so he could eventually start dating again. But he struggled to stay motivated and would fall off his habits. Eric's transformation rebuilt his body and his confidence so he could have another chance at love. Armed with his new body, and the tools to keep his motivation and habits going, he is confident and ready to start this new chapter of his life.
- **Diana, a 48-year-old doctor and mother of two.** During a period of high stress, Diana had gained weight and lost the mobility she needed to play sports with her kids. This left her feeling very sad, frustrated, and "not like herself." Thanks to learning what habits would transform her body best and how to fit them into her super-packed schedule, she lost 50 lb and gained back her fitness and mobility. Today, she goes skiing with her kids and is, in her words, "over the moon" with her transformation.

- **Steve, a 50-year-old retail furniture executive.** To cope with toxic relationships, Steve would turn to marijuana. This led to some other bad habits, like emotional eating. As a result, he gained weight and ended up with gut dysbiosis. He dreaded the idea that he was going to enter his fifties unhealthy and unhappy. Thanks to following our coaching on how to set boundaries and remove negative influences from his life, as well as on how to eat the right foods at the right times, Steve is 30 lb lighter, has improved digestion and is proud of his transformation.
- **Tracy, a 45-year-old corporate attorney and mother of two.** Remember Tracy? We met her at the beginning of the book. Her confidence at work and intimacy in the bedroom were affected by her 36% body fat and pre-diabetic A1C levels. Today she keeps her weight within 1–3 pounds of her target weight and has reduced her A1C to a healthy level. Tracy added significant muscle tone and also improved her strength by over 100%. Two years after completing *The Nine Shifts*, she emailed me a photo of her and her husband, Dylan, skiing together in the Alps.

Over the last five years, my team and I at my wellness practice, the InPowerment Company have been working very closely with our clients, all of them professionals over-40, to help them achieve a lasting, authentic transformation. I've gone deep into their situations, helping them work through the mental roadblocks that were holding them back from having the body they desired.

Together, we dove deep into their thought patterns, ingrained beliefs, and old identities that were formed years ago.

We also worked on any metabolic and hormonal obstacles such as high blood sugar, thyroid issues, low testosterone or gut health conditions. Combined with the other habits, tools and skills they've learned through *The Nine Shifts*, they have had remarkable results.

I'm particularly proud of the fact we've helped clients quit drinking habits, reduce usage of drugs (legal and illegal), and even restored their self-worth and confidence after losing a loved one or getting divorced. I'm proud to say that I've helped my clients understand themselves better and overcome mental challenges that had been ailing them for years.

Some of my clients have been through some very difficult experiences. Others, less so. But all of us have had, to one extent or another, our share of difficulties. Regardless of whether we've been through big traumas or small ones, we all have been shaped by the scars those experiences have left behind. These scars shape our personality and affect everything we do, including our emotions, confidence, self-worth, and our consistency.

By helping my clients become aware of their scars and teaching them how to reprogram their minds to create a more empowered, grounded, loving, peaceful, and confident version of themselves, everything has shifted for them, including their ability to stay consistent with habits that keep their mind, body, and life in the best place it can be.

Now let's talk about how you can, too.

CHAPTER 3

The First Step

"The first step toward success is taken when you refuse to be a captive of the environment in which you find yourself."
—Mark Caine

I've been talking a lot about transformations. For myself, for my clients, and now, for you. So, when I say that you, too, can have a lasting total transformation in your mind, body, and life, what exactly do I mean?

WHAT IT MEANS TO TRANSFORM

The word "transformation" is used very loosely these days. Some online coaches or health professionals promise to help you achieve a "body transformation" but what they're really referring to is losing body fat and gaining muscle—***temporarily***. You may have some success while they work with you and hold you accountable but the minute your program ends, your old thought patterns, identity, beliefs, and habits will return, and your old body will return with them.

When I say "transform," I'm not referring to following someone else's rules around dieting and exercise for a while to force your body to change, only to regress later. A true transformation is deeper than that—it's foundational and lasting. It involves going through a process to rewire your thoughts, identity, and beliefs through greater self-awareness and a reinvention of who you are at the most fundamental level. It results in tapping into deep sources of personal power that you can move mountains with, practicing routines that give you an unshakeable sense of calm, and releasing all of the old, outdated beliefs and ideas that can keep you stuck. It's about gaining self-awareness and the tools to release negative emotions like anxiety, depression, and boredom that can drive bad habits like emotional eating and other negative coping mechanisms. It's also about learning how to stay motivated and beat procrastination, even in the face of heavy work and life demands.

Transforming means to become the best version of yourself, from the inside out and from the ground up, so that you can't backslide, you can't revert and you can't be stopped. You have reconnected with ***who you really are***, and no one can take that away from you. In the process, you change everything: your mental habits and beliefs, your daily and weekly routines, and your environment.

Yes, that includes your body. We are talking about transforming your mind, your body, and your life, and the body is the main focus of the equation. Besides preventing you from being a lesser version of yourself, consider all the things that a fully healthy and fit body allows you to do:

- **Access greater energy and vitality**—You're more productive at work and at home, which is essential because, as *The Power of Full Engagement* teaches us, "energy, not time, is the fundamental currency of high performance."[11]
- **Carry yourself more confidently**—Nothing ensures success quite like exuding confidence in all your interactions.
- **Make better decisions**—A healthy body increases mental clarity and improves decision making.
- **Manage stress better**—Being self-aware and grounded helps you handle life's challenges better.
- **Age more gracefully and with greater freedom**—Do what you love into your advanced years while keeping aches and pains low.
- **Prevent illness**—Keep your immune system primed and limit illness from slowing you down.

I hope by now I've convinced you that this transformation is both essential and possible for you, and have inspired you to want to take your first step on the journey of transformation. If so, let's take a moment to find out where you are now.

WHERE ARE YOU STARTING FROM?

Management guru Peter Drucker is famous for saying "What gets measured gets improved." To that end, let's quickly set up a baseline to better understand where you're starting from and what aspects of your transformation to measure. We're just going to establish an easy, intuitive snapshot of where you are now, at this moment. It will help you along the way to remember what your personal transformation goals are, to remember why you're doing this when you're unsure, and give you a place to focus when you're overwhelmed. And then, after you've made some of the shifts in this book, the best part will be checking in to measure your progress against this initial baseline and see how far you've come.

To get a baseline of where you are now, choose an answer for each of the nine questions below with how closely

MIND

1. I stress eat with comfort foods, alcohol, or other substances at least once per week.
2. I feel burned out, overwhelmed, anxious, bored, or depressed at least once per week.
3. I feel my motivation level to eat healthy and exercise slipping after a few short weeks.

BODY

1. I struggle to lose weight even when I try my hardest to eat healthy and exercise.
2. I have insulin resistance, pre-diabetes, Type 2 diabetes, low testosterone, or have been through menopause.
3. I would describe my sleep as below average (i.e., I have more bad nights of sleep than good ones).

LIFE

1. I feel stressed out, angry, or get triggered at least once per week.
2. I struggle to find the time to do everything I need to do, including my own self-care.
3. I get thrown off my good health habits by things like travel, social events, or holidays.

you agree or disagree with the statement. (On scale of 1–10, where 1 is "Strongly Disagree" and 10 is "Strongly Agree.")

There is no right or wrong answer and no need to share this with anyone. This is just for you.

When you're finished, **add up your total score** from all the questions, and turn the page to see what your score likely means for you.

1	2	3	4	5	6	7	8	9	10	SCORE
○	○	○	○	○	○	○	○	○	○	
○	○	○	○	○	○	○	○	○	○	
○	○	○	○	○	○	○	○	○	○	

1	2	3	4	5	6	7	8	9	10	SCORE
○	○	○	○	○	○	○	○	○	○	
○	○	○	○	○	○	○	○	○	○	
○	○	○	○	○	○	○	○	○	○	

1	2	3	4	5	6	7	8	9	10	SCORE
○	○	○	○	○	○	○	○	○	○	
○	○	○	○	○	○	○	○	○	○	
○	○	○	○	○	○	○	○	○	○	

SCORE RESULTS

0–29

Mostly satisfied with your body, health, and life. Feeling in control but experiencing occasional self-doubt or setbacks. You know there is some room for improvement but are not totally motivated to make the sacrifices or are not sure how to get to that next level. Sometimes you wonder how to get more out of the time you're spending on your habits.

30–49

Habits and mindset are not amazing but not terrible either. Doing your best considering everything you're up against. Energy, health, and body are "OK." You sometimes wonder if you're maybe being complacent or stuck in your comfort zone.

50–69

Doing your best to do something versus nothing. Motivation comes and goes. Energy, habits, and overall health could be better. Concerned with what will happen if it gets harder to hold onto the minimum amount you're doing now.

70–90

Common challenges are frequently getting in the way. Health habits are being deprioritized for long stretches, causing low energy, excess body fat, and/or elevated health markers. Concerned about your quality of life and your future. Confidence and motivation are down while stress and unhappiness are an ongoing battle.

WHAT YOUR SCORE REALLY MEANS

Kind of like when you took the SAT (Scholastic Aptitude Test), (Do you remember that wonderful experience?) your score doesn't mean anything about you, personally. It's merely an indicator of how close or how far you currently are from being where you want to be in the categories of mind, body, and life. Whatever your starting point, trust that you're exactly where you were meant to be right now.

If you aren't happy with your current score, know that most people aren't, and most never will be. The fact you're reading this book means that you're committed to rising above the average and achieving your best self.

NINE CHALLENGES STANDING IN YOUR WAY

You're on the road to learning what it takes to achieve a lasting transformation, one that is personal to you, just like all of the stories you've heard so far. I wish I could say it's going to be a piece of cake, but there are some challenges in your way. In fact, I've identified nine major challenges that can stop you. We need to move these challenges out of your way so that you can go from where you are now to where you want to be—and stay there. Nearly all of the people I have worked with used to be hindered by several of these challenges when trying to drive meaningful change.

These nine challenges can be grouped neatly into the categories of mind, body, and life.

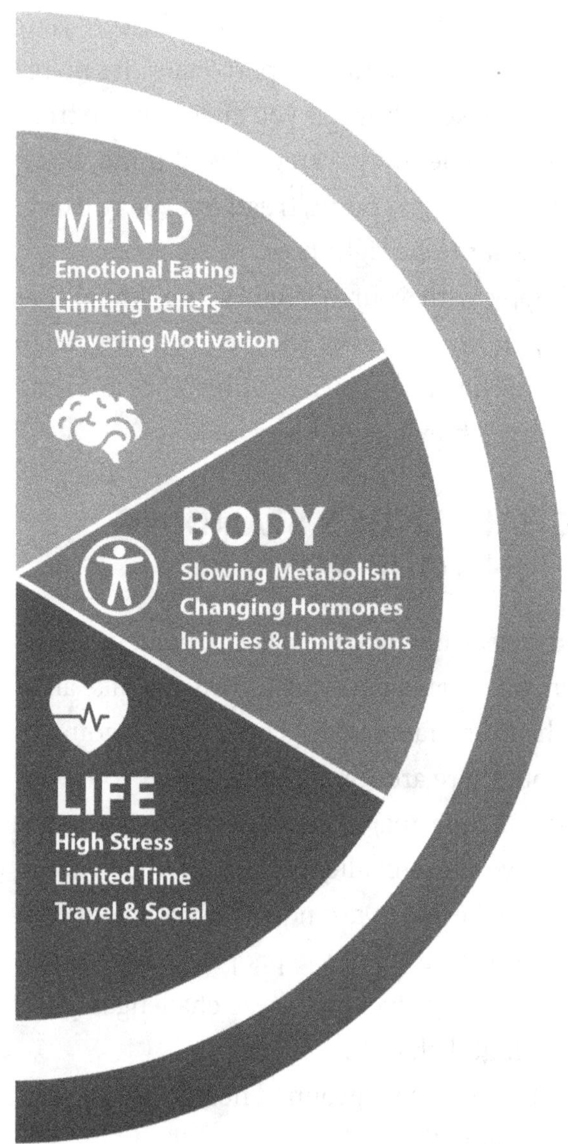
MIND
Emotional Eating
Limiting Beliefs
Wavering Motivation
BODY
Slowing Metabolism
Changing Hormones
Injuries & Limitations
LIFE
High Stress
Limited Time
Travel & Social

MIND

Mind-related challenges are the most important to conquer for long-term success because they can derail our ability to stay consistent with the habits that benefit our body. These challenges include:

1. Emotional eating often caused by internal stress or negative emotions
2. Limiting beliefs and identities such as perfectionism that cause us to overcompensate for perceived self-worth inadequacies (i.e., each one of our versions of "I'm not good enough")
3. Motivation swings caused by the fickle and distracted nature of our mind

BODY

Body-related challenges are caused by our stage of life and make it harder to lose body fat and build muscle tone. They include:

1. Metabolic decline due to age and lifestyle factors
2. Changing hormones due to life stage (such as menopause) and other disruptors such as medications, conditions, or illnesses
3. Injury risk or limitations due to age, weight, or prior injuries

LIFE

Life-related challenges can also derail us from our transformation goals. They include:

1. External stress from our jobs or relationship dynamics
2. Limited time due to the many responsibilities we carry
3. Travel and social events that cause interruptions and temptations of rich food or drink.

As we continue through this book, this framework—which you can think of as a speedometer—will help guide you. It will show you where you are on the path and indicate whether we're referring to the category of your mind, your body, or your life.

Are you ready to put the pedal to the metal and ***shift?***

A NOTE OF EMPATHY

Now, in case you're hesitant because you've struggled to achieve your body transformation goals in the past and this has caused you to lose hope, then let me prevent any chance of your mind going into Debbie Downer mode by sharing this bit of empathy with you:

Please know that there is no shame in struggling with one's body. You are definitely not alone.

Remember, it took me thirty years to achieve lasting change in my own body.

I vividly recall the days when I struggled, feeling stuck and frustrated.

It was no fun.

After coaching 120+ executives and high-achieving career professionals in achieving their transformation goals, I can tell you that even smart, successful people struggle with getting and maintaining results..

So take heart.

The answers are coming and the solutions are right around the corner.

EVEN THE TOUGHEST CASES

Working closely with each of my clients (some of whom you will read about throughout the book), and supporting them in adopting *The Nine Shifts*, led each person to achieve and maintain an incredible transformation, one that was personal to them. As you read through their stories in the last chapter, I hope you noticed something. Some of these people came to us with complications; this is common in midlife.

Health issues and disorders, such as hormonal imbalances, are not uncommon for those over forty. Walter came to us with Hashimoto's Disease (an autoimmune disease that depresses thyroid function) and was suffering from low testosterone. Tracy came to us with elevated A1C. Tammy came to us with post-menopausal, pre-diabetes, and anxiety medication usage.

While these issues made it harder for them to shed weight and build muscle, our system and support are designed to help you overcome them, even if these things have made it harder in the past to reach your goals.

This book will give you the clear, proven steps to take in order to look, feel, and perform your best. However, certain physiological or psychological complications can make it harder to get results, even with a proven process.

If you're struggling to achieve your transformation goals, whether due to health issues, a lack of time, overwhelm, limited motivation, confusion about what works best, or some other challenge, know this: ***my team and I are here for you***.

Because we specialize in an over-40 population, advising you on blood work and health markers is an important aspect of how we design your personalized *Nine Shifts* transformation program. In fact, we partner with a full team of advisors, including functional medicine doctors, metabolism experts, dietitians, labs, and mental health practitioners, in order to address the most complex cases.

Sometimes, it takes deeper expertise and some ongoing support to overcome complications and create the breakthrough in your body that you've been seeking. The typical advice of "just eat less and move more" doesn't always work, especially as we get older (later in this book, you'll see why that is).

MY INVITATION

To learn more about how we can support you to overcome complications that might be causing you to struggle making progress, feel free to apply for a complimentary Breakthrough Call via this link: https://thenineshifts.com/call

PART II
The Challenges

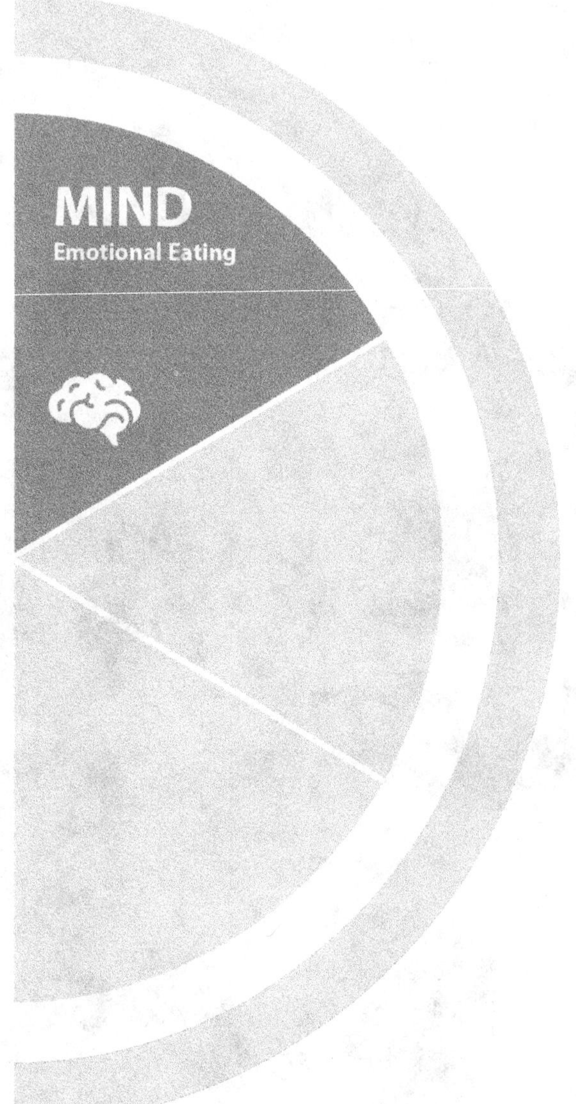
MIND
Emotional Eating

CHAPTER 4

CHALLENGE #1: Emotional Eating

"Emotion can be the enemy, if you give into your emotion, you lose yourself. You must be at one with your emotions, because the body always follows the mind."
—Bruce Lee

I like to say, "A stressful day never met a pint of ice cream it didn't love." In fact, drowning our emotions in a tub of rocky road (or a bottle of Merlot) is pretty common. According to the American Psychological Association, close to 40% percent of U.S. adults overeat or make unhealthy food choices each month because of stress. Half of those adults said they do it weekly.[12]

It's become so common that it's sort of a given for most people to numb the pain of stress or other negative emotions with comfort foods and other vices.

- Stressful day at work? We wash it away with wine.
- Feeling down about ourselves? Sweet treats to ease the pain.
- Anxious about the future? There's always a pill (or drug) for that.

When we lack tools and awareness to cope with emotional stress, it can set us back in our health habits. My client, Brooke, told me on one of our coaching calls that she had a "bad week." When I asked her what happened, she said she had found out her ex-husband (who she still had regular contact with due to their custody agreement for their children) had started seeing a younger woman. It cut Brooke to the bone and triggered her limiting beliefs about herself; that she was too old, too unattractive, too worthless to be able to have a loving relationship. Understandably, this hit her hard—and she spent the next three days lying in bed and eating comfort foods.

Following her meal plan or getting some movement in went straight out the window.

Numbing our emotions has become so normal that most of us accept it without question. And don't get me wrong, I knew Brooke was in pain and needed some extra TLC. But I ***also*** knew that if she was going to be consistent, she needed to develop the skill to snap out of these negative states quickly—in three minutes, not three days!

What makes this challenge so difficult is the fact that it's a natural, human reaction to want to soothe ourselves when we feel emotional pain. To not let negative emotions derail you, the goal is to become aware of how your thoughts and emotions are driving your actions, so that you can be in charge of your thoughts, instead of them being in charge of you.

I will confess that I struggled with anxiety for many years. Throughout my twenties and early thirties I would often feel anxious, experience heart palpitations, and feel like time was running out on me—that the walls were closing in. Anytime I'd be late for something or have to rush to catch a subway (I was living in NYC at the time) or a flight (I traveled a lot for work) my anxiety would go through the roof and it would take a long time to bring my internal state back to normal.

It wasn't until I started doing deep transformation and personal development work in my mid-thirties that I was able to get to the root of my anxiety by healing past traumas, rewiring my limiting beliefs, and getting a better grasp of how the mind works. I'd like to help you do the same because stress, anxiety, worry, and depression are part of the human experience and they cause suffering. In turn, these feelings can drive us to crave things like processed foods or alcohol more often than is ideal. But with the right tools we can begin to gain power over our mind, our thoughts, and our emotions. This will lead to greater peace, clarity, and consistency in our habits, including our body transformation habits.

EMOTIONS ARE DRIVING THE BUS

Humans are emotional beings. Our emotions are a core part of who we are and they influence our actions a lot more than logic does. In fact, some studies have shown that up to 90% of the decisions we make are primarily influenced by our emotions.[13] If this is true, then it means emotions can influence almost all of the actions we take—or don't take—towards achieving the body and health we desire.

Real change doesn't come from hearing logical advice. It comes from learning how to better understand and manage our emotions.

Smokers know that smoking is bad for them. There's no logical reason to smoke, yet they continue to light up because it makes them feel good.

No one needs to spend $250,000 on a car when they can spend $25,000. There's no logical reason to spend ten times more. But people ***do*** spend ten times more because driving a Bentley makes them feel better than driving a Honda.

If logic doesn't really work to create change, how do we tap into our emotions to create the changes we seek?

EVERY EMOTION STARTS WITH A THOUGHT

Our emotions come from our thoughts. Think of something happy, you feel happy. Think of something sad, you feel sad, and so on. The actions we take are based on the combination of our thoughts and our feelings. If we want our actions to get us closer to our goal then our thoughts and feelings have to align with each other, and with our goal.

If I have a logical thought that says "I should workout tonight" but my feeling about that thought is "I don't feel like it," there's a pretty good chance the action isn't happening—I'll probably skip my workout tonight.

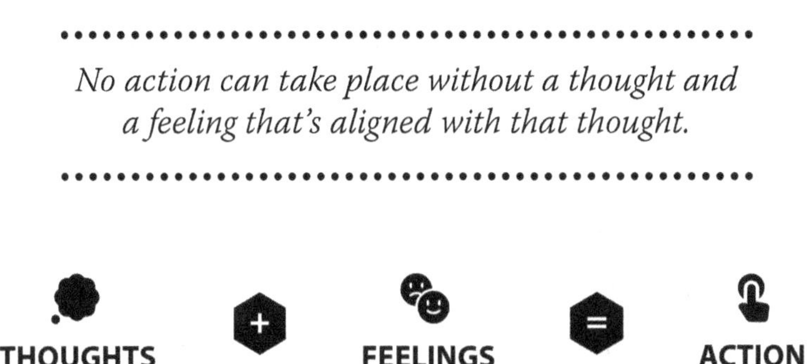

No action can take place without a thought and a feeling that's aligned with that thought.

Scientists estimate that humans have 70,000 thoughts per day.[14] Most of these are negative, fear-based thoughts driven by a survival-focused mind that was handed down to us from our ancestors who constantly had to worry about threats like not having enough food, being attacked by predators, and even war.

What makes things particularly challenging is the fact our thoughts feel like they are us. Except they're not.

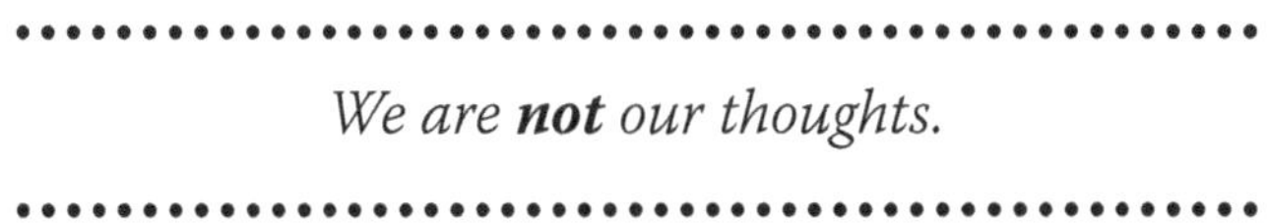

*We are **not** our thoughts.*

In its quest to protect us, part of the mind's design is its ability to convince us that our thoughts are who we are. Because of this sneaky construct, the mind keeps most people in constant reactionary mode, obeying the thoughts of the mind and the feelings they bring forth.

- Didn't land that dream job you were eager to get? The mind feels like a failure, worries that we're unworthy, and we feel depressed.

- Saw someone at the gym who has the type of body you'd kill for? The mind goes into comparison mode, feels like we don't add up, and never will, and we feel hopeless.
- Need to give a speech? The mind worries that you will make a goof of yourself in a public setting. This triggers deep-seated fears that our tribe will reject us and that we don't fit in, so it starts to feel anxious.

This plethora of negative thoughts lead to negative emotions. In turn, negative emotions can lead to behaviors that are incongruent with our body transformation goals, such as stress eating, stress drinking, and skipping workouts.

WHY WE STRESS EAT

When we feel negative emotions such as stress, anger, depression, boredom, or anxiety, our natural instinct is to quickly eliminate those feelings. That's because our mind is wired to move away from pain and toward pleasure. Upon feeling these negative emotions, the mind will push you to find ways to numb or cancel out those feelings via different coping mechanisms. Everyone's coping mechanisms are different and can include anything from comfort food and binging on television to alcohol or drugs.

This can happen even if we "know better." (Again, it's not about what's logical.) You know how sometimes our emotions get the best of us during an argument and we say something we later regret? Well, sometimes we do the same thing with food. Our emotions get the best of us and we eat or drink something we'll later regret. We stress eat.

Any number of things can send us into an emotional tailspin. If we don't have a solid plan in place to manage our thoughts and emotions, it's very likely that our mind will derail us. Stressful days turn into stressful weeks, stressful weeks turn into stressful months, and ongoing stressful situations, like a toxic work environment or relationship, keep us in constant survival mode.

THERE'S HOPE FOR EMOTIONAL EATING

If you've been struggling with emotional eating or cravings and it's affected your body and health negatively, it's important to address your emotions directly. This will give you the best chance of becoming lean, staying healthy, and being happy overall. While choosing better coping mechanisms can help (like carrot sticks instead of potato chips), they're more of a band aid and only treat the symptom.

By gaining mastery over your mind and your emotions, you will create the right environment for the body to thrive. Not only will you reduce chronic stress, which (as you will learn shortly) can lead to elevated cortisol levels and many nasty adaptations like elevated blood sugar and inflammation that can hinder your body transformation goals, but you'll also prevent negative emotions from wrecking your day and derailing your health habits in the process. You'll learn how to make this shift in Chapter 15, "Shift #1: Master Your Emotions." In the meantime, I'll leave you with a quick action that you can start doing now to gain more power over your emotions and any stress eating challenges you're encountering.

At the end of each of the challenge chapters I'm going to give you something you can do immediately—a quick action. We'll go over the complete solution in Part III, but in the meantime, I encourage you to experiment with the mini-activity at the end of each challenge chapter, starting with the one that follows.

QUICK ACTION

An easy but powerful way to shift out of negative emotions that can lead to stress eating is simply to give gratitude. At a metaphysical level, feeling grateful is a soul-based vibrational energy which is more powerful than lower level energies like anxiety, depression, jealousy, sadness, or fear. When we're feeling gratitude we're immune to feeling those negative states of the mind. Counting your blessings really works. As the American author Zig Ziglar said "Of all the 'attitudes' we can acquire, surely the attitude of gratitude is the most important and by far the most life-changing."

So go ahead. Answer any of these three gratitude-based questions below and see how quickly they shift you into a positive state:

- What am I grateful for today?
- Who am I grateful for today?
- In what way am I blessed today?

Feeling better? Great!

Use them anytime you're feeling off.

In fact, you can use them ***all*** of the time. Watch how staying present to them helps you start attracting more of what you're grateful for.

FORMER AIRLINE INDUSTRY EXEC LEARNS TO STAY MOTIVATED AND SOARS TO A SIX-PACK AT 65

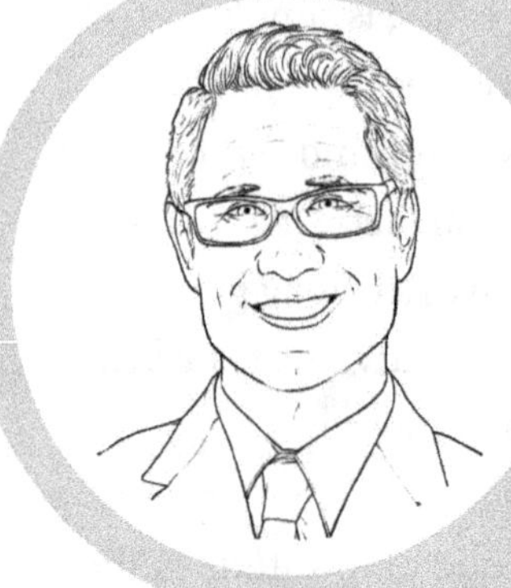

This program is very concise. You've given me the tools I need. You give the truth about what it's going to take. Incredible nutrition and supplementation and the chemistry behind that. –Eric

THE SITUATION

Eric's partner had been struck and killed by a car while jogging one night near their home. Once he took time to fully process the grief of this loss, he felt ready to start the next chapter of his life. He wanted to regain his confidence so he could eventually start dating again.

Even though he had reached retirement age and had a slower metabolism, Eric didn't have a lot of weight to lose. Nevertheless, he felt "soft" and not in his best shape. He wanted to firm up and shed some belly fat. Eric was committed to looking and feeling his best.

Eric tried working with a personal trainer but would regress every time he'd stop. His motivation to continue on his own simply wavered without the support of his personal trainer. He also got set back by weekend potluck dinners with his social circle of friends. There was so much pressure to indulge in rich food and drink at these events that he just couldn't resist.

THE SOLUTION

We started by teaching Eric mindset techniques for generating motivation without relying on others. We also gave Eric a flexible nutrition strategy that would allow him to balance getting the fat down while still enjoying the weekend gatherings with his friends. Experimenting with several nutritional strategies, we found one that would suit his preferences and fit his lifestyle best. We also added new approaches to his strength and cardio training that he had not yet tried. These techniques allowed him to build more muscle tone and burn more fat than ever before.

THE TRANSFORMATION

By implementing the tools and techniques we provided, Eric started to make consistent progress in transforming his body, successfully adding muscle tone and reducing belly fat. Very soon his chest became less saggy, his midsection more tight, and his posture noticeably improved. At the age of sixty-five, he was able to attain a six-pack and a more chiseled body.

"Efficiency and time management are very important to me. This program is very concise. You've given me the tools I need. You give the 'truth' about what it's going to take. Incredible nutrition and supplementation and the chemistry behind that. Plus, the mindset. It all works together. My physique has changed. I can see it. I feel great, I really do."

The fact that Eric achieved his body transformation goals while still enjoying his weekend group outings was a definite win in his opinion. Achieving the results at his age would have been out of reach for most sixty-five year olds. He credits his transformation to us helping him gain the confidence to start dating again so he can have another chance at love.

MIND

Emotional Eating

Limiting Beliefs

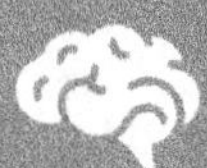

CHAPTER 5

CHALLENGE #2: Limiting Beliefs

"You can't escape from a prison until
you recognize you are in one."
—Bob Proctor

As humans, beliefs drive our decisions. If I believe that the world is flat I will avoid sailing too close to the edge of the earth. In this case, even though the belief is actually not true (the world is not flat) it acts to influence my decisions and will limit how far I can travel.

Beliefs that can hinder our results and prevent us from reaching our fullest potential are called limiting beliefs. *"A limiting belief is a thought or state of mind that you think is the absolute truth and stops you from doing certain things. These beliefs don't always have to be about yourself, either. They could be about how the world works . . . "*[15]

When it comes to transforming our bodies, there are two types of limiting beliefs that can impede our progress:

- Beliefs about who we are.
- Beliefs about what is or is not possible for us to accomplish.

The first type of limiting belief is a fear-based view of one's self. It shapes how we see ourselves and influences our identity—who we are. It encapsulates how we see our own self-worth. I call this our Core Limiting Belief.

The second type of limiting belief is also driven by fear and shows up as flaws in our thinking about what's possible. As you will see, these two types of limiting beliefs make it harder to keep our bodies where we want them.

Now, I realize that digging into our beliefs can be pretty deep stuff. So let me unpack this topic a bit to make sure it's clear. First, we will go over what a limiting belief is and how it works. Second, you will see how your limiting beliefs are formed by the mind in its quest to ensure your survival, and how these limiting beliefs influence your identity. Third, you will see how that identity (which is actually based on a lie) makes us overcompensate and act in ways that cause us to lose our balance and procrastinate on our health goals. Later, in Chapter 16, you will learn how to transform your limiting beliefs and recreate yourself as a new, more empowered identity that's free from the imaginary shackles that are created by those limiting beliefs.

HOW LIMITING BELIEFS WORK

If, deep down, we have a fear-based belief that stops us from taking the actions that will lead to the outcomes that we want, we will procrastinate and we will struggle in that area.

This can apply to relationships, as one example. Endure a heartbreak and you're less likely to fall in love again. What may surprise you is that the reason the heartbreak hurt so bad is not because your heart broke into pieces (that's just a figure of speech, of course) but because it triggered your core limiting belief; you just didn't know it.

Needless to say, this can also apply to our body transformation goals. For example, my client Ingrid, due to childhood abuse she had endured, was harboring a fear-based belief of "I don't matter." This negative (and untrue) belief about her self-worth would cause her to eat poorly because, per this belief, whether she's healthy or not doesn't matter either.

Our core limiting belief usually begins at a young age as our personalities are developing, and it is usually hidden from our view. We believe the belief to be true, and it shapes how we see ourselves, and plays a role in forming our personality. Operating with this belief for years and even decades, it becomes part of how we interact with the world, and if it's ever questioned, we usually explain it away as just being part of our personality—"It's how I've always been."

HOW CORE LIMITING BELIEF AND IDENTITY BEGIN (THE TRAUMA CHAIN)

One of the mind's survival tactics is seeking to win the favor and acceptance of others, namely our parents and our tribe, to ensure that they protect us as we're growing up. If the mind senses that we are not winning their love and acceptance, it will come up with alternative strategies to win them over.

The mind's objective is to help us survive and will do anything, including tell us lies, to ensure our survival.

To understand how our limiting beliefs and identity get started, we can observe what I call "The Trauma Chain" in the diagram below:

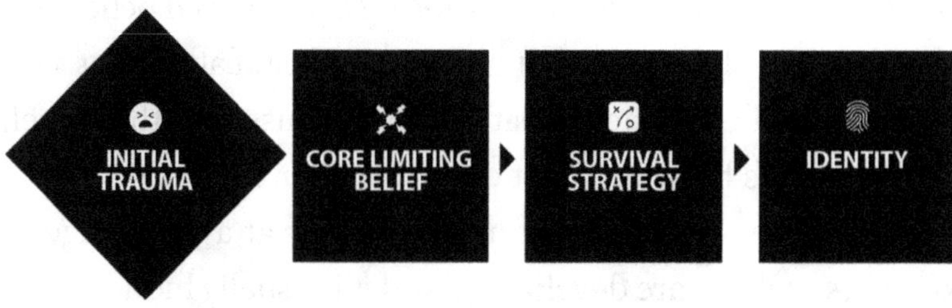

It is believed that our core limiting belief is usually formed when we experience our first trauma as children, usually between the ages of three and seven. This initial trauma—be it large or small—goes unresolved and makes us believe that our trust has been broken, and makes us feel unsafe, unloved, unworthy, and unprotected. The young mind senses this, and because it's not fully developed from an emotional or maturity standpoint yet, the mind interprets incorrectly that there must be something wrong with us. We must lack self-worth. Therefore, we must have some kind of inadequacy.

The inadequacy we believe to be true about ourselves creates our core limiting belief. For example, if a child is teased at school for a bad grade they received, he or she may conclude, "I don't belong."

Given this perceived flaw (which is untrue), the child subconsciously fears rejection by those around him. The child decides that he or she needs to compensate for this flaw in order to win back the acceptance and protection of others.

HOW OUR LIMITING BELIEF CREATES OVERCOMPENSATION AND FORMS OUR IDENTITY

To make up for their perceived inadequacy, and feel worthy of the love and protection of his or her classmates (their tribe), the child's mind devises a survival strategy. For example, "I need to be *perfect* with my grades from this point forward in order to feel like I belong and am accepted." Operating from our survival strategy in order to fill the void in our self-worth, that's created by the limiting belief, creates our identity. For example we might become a "Perfectionist."

Many of my clients are high achievers. A large majority of them (myself included) have a limiting belief around perfectionism. Perfectionism can stem from trying to win favor of parents or those around them through accomplishments. This learned behavior results in driving themselves hard, setting very high or unrealistic standards for themselves, and, when it comes to improving their bodies, going to extremes with their diets or their exercise. But if their schedule doesn't allow them to get in the perfect workout they abandon the idea completely and do nothing instead of doing a workout that doesn't meet their high standards. This results in an "all-in/all-out" approach to their habits that sabotages their consistency.

Your core limiting belief, and the identity it saddles you with, comes from a misinterpretation of a traumatic event you experienced as a child.

Because the originating trauma leaves a deep emotional scar and results in intense fear and negative feelings it creates strong neural connections in the mind. This creates subconscious patterns that stay with us, and that we keep repeating. The more we repeat them, the more they get reinforced and become habitual loops that become our fixed ways of being—our identity.

Limiting beliefs can run the gamut of self-doubts and have us playing what I call the "What if Game." It leads us to ask fear-based questions such as: "What if I'm not good enough?", "What if I'm not doing this right?", or "What if no one loves me?" These beliefs can cause us to feel anxious, doubt ourselves, and even lead to impostor syndrome.

As another example of how identity is formed, consider a child that is experiencing physical abuse. As he or she goes through that trauma and tries to understand what's happening, they might begin to believe, "I'm unworthy of love." When that child becomes an adult, they might compensate for this feeling of unworthiness by being overly compliant and never saying no, in order to attain the love they're afraid of missing out on. It's almost as if a part of them is still trying to avoid upsetting their childhood era abuser in order to win their acceptance. By subconsciously trying to protect themselves in this way, the limiting belief caused them to take on the identity of a "People Pleaser."

This identity is focused on making those around us constantly happy. This feeds the people pleaser's self-worth. It also prevents them from upsetting others in order to avoid triggering prior feelings of pain from abuse, rejection, or retribution. However, because it comes from a pretense, this identity of having to always please others in order to feel accepted and worthy can make us apprehensive to speak up and ask for what we truly want and need.

In this way, this identity can preclude the person from saying "no" and setting a healthy boundary that serves to protect their time, including the time they need for completing their body transformation habits. People pleasers are notorious for always being overwhelmed.

Limiting beliefs about who we are can lead to overcompensating for the subconscious fears of feeling unworthy in a way that makes it harder to maintain our transformation habits. (More on how this works in Chapter 14, "Mindset 101.")

The subconscious need to win acceptance by being perfect or pleasing others can lead to burn out or overwhelm, both of which can hinder our body transformation habits.

Let's look at some of the more common fear-based identities to show how they can make it harder to stay consistent with our body transformation habits. The list is not exhaustive but it includes some of the most common ones I've noticed in working with clients.

Identity	Limiting Belief	Challenge to Body Goals
The Perfectionist	"I need to be perfect and earn acceptance and validation through my achievements."	Going to extremes with diet and training. All-in/all-out streaks of major motivation or completely throwing in the towel.
The People Pleaser	"I can't say no or people won't love me."	Lack of boundaries which leads to a lack of time, overwhelm, losing balance, and losing sight of health goals.
The Victim	"Things happen ***to*** me. I'm trapped and powerless to change them."	Self-fulfilling prophecy that the world is out to get you and that you can't catch a break. Self-doubt in your ability to achieve your goals.
The Sacrificial Lamb	"I can't trust others and need to do it all myself."	Overwhelm, stress, lack of life satisfaction, very long to-do list which seems to never get done. Delegating and asking for help is a real struggle. Constant worry and limited time to do things for oneself, including self-care.

Now, ask yourself these questions:

- Did you find yourself on that list?
- Can you relate to some of these limiting beliefs?
- Can you see how they may have shaped your identity?
- Is there a different identity that's not on this list with which you identify?

Again, this list is not exhaustive, you may have another identity. This list is also not mutually exclusive; you may relate to more than one of these identities and perhaps you toggle between them. (Personally, I've fluctuated between being a Perfectionist and a People Pleaser.)

Whichever identity we take on, if it's based on a limiting belief, it can throw us off track when it comes to balancing our day-to-day lives and keeping a balance with our health. Worse still, is the fact our mind will make up excuses and justify inaction in order to keep the survival-based identity in place. The mind will say things like, "It's OK, you can just work out another day" to prevent the People Pleaser from telling the boss they can't work late again. It may say "As soon as things slow down, I'll get back into my routine" to keep the Perfectionist working hard to keep earning money or accolades.

Of course, staying late at work or hustling to get ahead are sometimes required. But if they are continuously preventing us from spending time on our health habits and self-care, then they may be coming from a place of fear—our core limiting belief, and will cause us to eventually become unhealthy; this is not sustainable.

Here are some examples from some of my own clients.

Client	Core Limiting Belief	Survival Strategy
Nadine	"I'm not worth it."	Be nice and never say "no."
Michael	"I'm irrelevant."	Need to work hard and prove myself.
Ingrid	"I don't matter."	Need to be strong and support everyone else.

In those client examples above, we see how each person's survival strategy causes overcompensation for the mind's perceived lack of self-worth. To make matters worse, the identity they've taken on causes resistance to take any action at all, leading to procrastination.

Again, some of us endure smaller traumas, while others endure bigger ones. I've heard some difficult stories about abuses and tragedies that some of my clients went through and my heart breaks every time I hear them. It's why I feel so blessed to have grown up in a household that was full of peace and love. My parents, two amazingly loving and strong

Identity	Imbalance
People Pleaser	Stays late at work and takes extra shifts to help coworkers; enters toxic relationships where the other continuously takes; rarely says "no" or sets boundaries; has little to no time or energy left for a health routine.
Perfectionist	Works hard in business; doesn't have help; misses workouts; gets down; does nothing the rest of the week; waits until next week (all-in/all-out).
Sacrificial Lamb	Always puts everyone else's needs first; gets exhausted; rarely has time or energy left for self-care.

parents (and now grandparents), properly loved, nurtured, and educated my younger brother and I, instilling the values and discipline needed for us to grow up to be upstanding members of society.

HOW MY CORE LIMITING BELIEF SHAPED ME

Thankfully, my originating trauma was a minor one. But like for most of us, it happened at a tender time and left a scar, which shaped my identity. My core limiting belief is that "I'm weak." It happened the first time I was disciplined by my parents at the age of five (I totally deserved it, lol). I actually had completely forgotten about the event until I was sitting in one of my transformation courses and we did an exercise that took me back to that early memory. As a naive, scared child in pain, this was the incorrect conclusion I came up with that shaped my personality. My survival strategy was to be "compliant" and never upset anyone ever again so that I don't feel that level of intense hurt ever again.

So growing up, my subconscious fears would arise whenever I'd be interacting with someone who I'd perceive as either an authority figure or someone who seemed stronger than me or could hurt me: a bully at school, a bossy girlfriend, or my supervisor at work. I'd vacillate between being a Perfectionist and a People Pleaser to avoid getting hurt again. In hindsight, I think my limiting belief is what drove me to be the first of all my friends to start bodybuilding at the age of thirteen. Think about it: if you subconsciously fear that you're weak, what better way to compensate for that fear than by having muscles and appearing strong? (Pretty wild, right?)

Regardless of the size or duration of the traumas we endure, the scar is formed and the limiting belief distorts our vision of the world, totally unbeknownst to ourselves.

But if we want to be free of it, so that it does not cause us to overcompensate and lose sight of the habits that will keep our body and health where we want them, we must uncover our limiting belief, bring it to the light, heal it and transform it. Only by doing this will we become free. It's how I broke through, and how you will too.

You'll see how to break free in Chapter 16, "Shift #2: Rewire Limiting Beliefs."

LIMITING BELIEFS ABOUT WHAT'S POSSIBLE

The other type of limiting belief to watch out for is when we make assumptions or draw conclusions based on limited information or fear-based justifications for our shortcomings. You may have heard some of these before (I hear them all the time). Examples include statements such as:

- "I'm too old to have the body I want."
- "I'm destined to be overweight because my entire family is fat."
- "I'm pretty sure my metabolism is frozen."

I would hear another common one from my client Edward, owner of a general contractor business. Any time he'd have a busy week and fall off of his transformation routine he'd lament, "My life is too crazy to focus on my health right now." (Sure, sir, whatever you say.)

These types of fear-based conclusions are based on subconscious fears and they justify our failure. They help us feel better about ourselves for not reaching the goal, even though deep down, we know we want it.

That was me, too, for many years. Even though I'd train hard in the gym and try to achieve my best body, any time I'd see a guy with a body way better than mine, I'd justify it by saying *"I'm juggling a lot of things right now. Besides, I'm sure that guy hasn't traveled to as many countries as I have."*

Clearly, these assumptions were justification my mind would come up with to make me feel better about being inferior in that area. They weren't based on fact. In reality, I had no idea how much that guy was juggling or how many countries he had been to. It was total BS—my mind's BS.

Even though these limiting beliefs would make me feel better temporarily, there was no getting around the fact my body wasn't where I wanted it to be. Ironically, that little bit of temporary relief these types of justifications give us release dopamine, which makes us feel better, and increases the chances we'll say the same thing when we're faced with another dose of reality the next time. This, in turn, increases the likelihood of not changing anything. As you can see, our minds are adept at covertly sabotaging us in order to keep us from feeling hurt and unworthy, but they also keep us—STUCK!

Here are some common limiting beliefs and assumptions around what's possible that can affect your body transformation goals:

- "I don't have enough time."
- "I'm too old to change (my body)."
- "My metabolism is broken."
- "I can't figure this out."
- "Losing weight will fix all my problems."
- "My life is too crazy to worry about myself, or my health."
- "I can't have it all." (i.e., either/or mentality. "Either I have a successful career or my desired body.")

Were you able to relate to some of these above? Can you think of some other limiting beliefs you tell yourself that aren't true but justify staying stuck where you are with your body and health?

In order to change the body, we must first change the mind.

THERE'S HOPE FOR LIMITING BELIEFS

The good news is that by rewiring your mind and taking on a more empowering identity, you will not only greatly improve your chances of having the health and body you want, but also improve the quality of your life overall. You will be happier, more calm, and more clear. You will get triggered less, worry less, and recover faster from negative states.

Your interpersonal relationships will improve because you will be more courageous in setting boundaries and asking for what you need. You will love more freely and express that love to those who matter to you most. More importantly, you will love yourself more, which will allow you to be more forgiving with yourself and others. You will become a source of joy for those around you.

You will start attracting more quality people into your life and you will not be scared to invite them into your circle. You will make deeper and more meaningful connections because you will be more at ease with who you are and the approval of others will no longer matter very much.

You will become more financially successful, because you'll have more guts to ask for that sale, request that raise, or go for that job. Moreover, you won't rely on shopping sprees, buying useless stuff, or paying needless markups to help deal with feelings of unworthiness.

For our purposes, you will not let negative emotions get the best of you and cause you to overcompensate by working too hard to prove yourself or to please others at the expense of your body and health goals.

Believe it or not, this is just a short list of what's possible when you learn how the mind works and get it working in your favor. If all this sounds too good to be true, it's not. These are all the amazing, powerful benefits I get to enjoy now that I've gone through a true mindset transformation. This is what awaits you, too, my friend, when you get to the top of the mountain.

Let me pull you up.

QUICK ACTION

To help uncover any limiting beliefs holding you back from making progress with your body and health, make a list of some beliefs you have about these areas. If you are struggling, you most likely have a limiting belief that's causing you to be stuck.

For example, if you believe that you don't have enough time to exercise, explore your limiting beliefs around time, in general, as well as how those beliefs apply to finding time to exercise. List out a few of these beliefs and start thinking about creative ways you can overcome the limitation they're placing on you. Make a list of all the things you spend your time on each week. Then see what you can cut, deprioritize, automate, or delegate to find yourself more time. (The Sacrificial Lambs will struggle with this the most because they hate asking for help. You guys may have to concentrate twice as hard for this exercise!)

Ultimately, get creative and think outside the box. Pretend like your life depends on you finding the solution to overcome your limiting beliefs. Because, in a very real sense, it does.

FAITH DROPS PERFECTIONISM AND GIVES EMOTIONAL EATING THE PINK SLIP

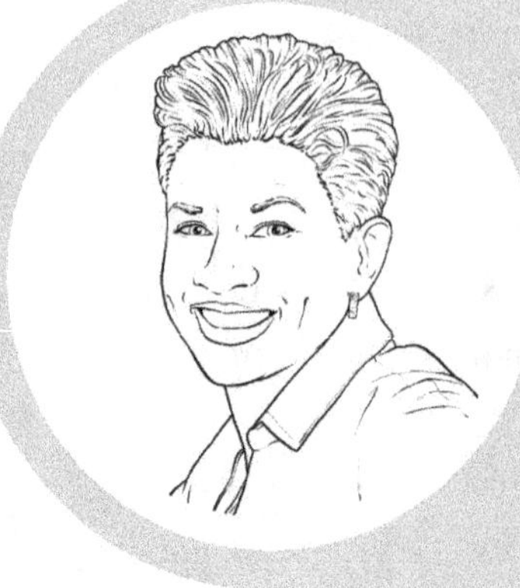

Before, I'd have a lot of highs and lows. When the emotions take over, that's when I overeat. But now, I consistently feel more balanced and don't get as overwhelmed.
–Faith

THE SITUATION

Faith truly embodied The Perfectionist identity. It started at an early age when she was exposed to the constant fighting of her parents and their eventual divorce—a very traumatic event. As a young child, she felt responsible for their fighting and tried to do her best to please her parents by being "perfect" and not making things between them worse.

As an adult, this identity of having to be perfect all the time would have her frequently take on a lot of work responsibilities to prove herself to her boss and her peers. This led to periods of overwhelm, then stress, and then emotional eating. Periods such as these would drive her weight up.

This would go on until the feelings of guilt got to be too much and her clothes started getting too tight. Then, she'd go the other extreme and try to be perfect with diet and exercise to lose the weight. Faith would be good for a while, until another bout of stress would hit and she'd start stress eating again.

It was a constant yo-yo in her habits and in her weight.

THE SOLUTION

Through the mindset work we did with Faith, we helped her uncover her old identity—"I have to be perfect." This took some deep work because our identities are ingrained subconsciously and are hidden from view. We explain them away as just part of our personality. "I've always been this way."

Once we uncovered that Faith's perfectionism was driving the overwhelm, we gave her tools to shift these thoughts and emotions. We taught her to be more aware of when she was acting from a need to prove herself so that she could give herself permission to decline extra work, speak up more, and ask for more resources, and staff. Faith was now able to release the impulse to have to prove herself by taking on a ton of work all the time.

Reducing the need to overcompensate by being perfect provided Faith with more spare time and energy to focus on self-care and doing her workouts more regularly. It also diminished her stress levels and greatly reduced her emotional eating.

THE TRANSFORMATION

Today, Faith is extremely proud to say she keeps her weight steady, no matter how busy or stressful things get.

"Before, I'd have a lot of highs and lows. When the emotions take over, that's when I overeat. But now, I consistently feel more balanced and don't get as overwhelmed. Seeing the impact of this mindset work on me blows me away!"

MIND

Emotional Eating

Limiting Beliefs

Wavering Motivation

CHAPTER 6

CHALLENGE #3: Wavering Motivation

"Don't stop until you're proud."
—Unknown

Got motivation?

No?

You're not alone.

When it comes to reaching one's body transformation goals, struggling to get motivated is a fairly common challenge. An article in *The Washington Post* called "Too Tired To Be Healthy," cites a survey that revealed nearly 40% of U.S. adults lacked motivation to be healthier.[16]

In my own unofficial estimates, two out of three prospects I speak with cite a lack of motivation as a key reason for their body struggles. Even some of my most successful clients, who are disciplined, high achieving career professionals like lawyers, bankers, and doctors, experience lapses in motivation.

What I have seen in my research and experience coaching clients is that most people struggle with motivation for two primary reasons:

1. They either wait around to feel motivated or rely on finite willpower.
2. They believe myths about motivation that cause them to make mistakes when trying to stay motivated.

Let's talk about both.

WHEN MOTIVATION FADES PEOPLE WAVER BETWEEN WAITING OR RELYING ON WILLPOWER

Not feeling motivated can dampen our spirits, make us feel deflated, and stop us from being in action around our goals. Simply put, it's hard to do hard things when we don't feel like doing them. We can only diet, exercise, or follow a program for so long if our motivation level tanks.

When it comes to drumming up the motivation to make a change in their body, most people start off with a certain level of excitement toward achieving their goal (e.g., lose 20 lb). Things generally go well at the beginning. They stay consistent with some habits and start to feel good.

But after a few weeks, the excitement fades, boredom starts to set it, and life throws challenges their way (e.g., a deadline at work, a trip, or a family event). So, they start to skip their workouts or are unable to stick to their restrictive diet. Lacking a proven plan, proper support, and the right knowledge about how to eat, train, and keep themselves motivated, they start to lose steam.

Their willpower is not strong enough and does not last long enough to overcome the obstacles. So they fall off their groove, lose their progress, become demotivated, and end up staying stuck. They usually stay idle here, or worse, regress. This goes on until a "triggering event" happens, such as being shocked at how they look in a photo, feeling dejected after receiving a critical remark about their body, or getting a scary lab result on their annual check up.

From a mindset perspective, what this event actually triggers is their core limiting belief of not being good enough, or it triggers fears of a bleak and unhealthy future. Both of these are painful feelings, and pain gets us to act. Except in this case, we're acting from a place of fear.

Driven by fear, they become desperate to get on track again. They do their best to muster up the willpower to resume their diet, track their calories, and start going to the gym again. Basically, they start this fruitless cycle all over.

I like to say that when it comes to trying to make a change in their body, most people are usually in one of two modes: using willpower or waiting for motivation to return.

People waver between two modes:
"Willpower" or "Waiting"

In the graph on the next page, you can see how fluctuating between these two modes results in their motivation level following an extreme up and down pattern of a rollercoaster. Not surprisingly, their body weight usually follows suit, in lock-step.

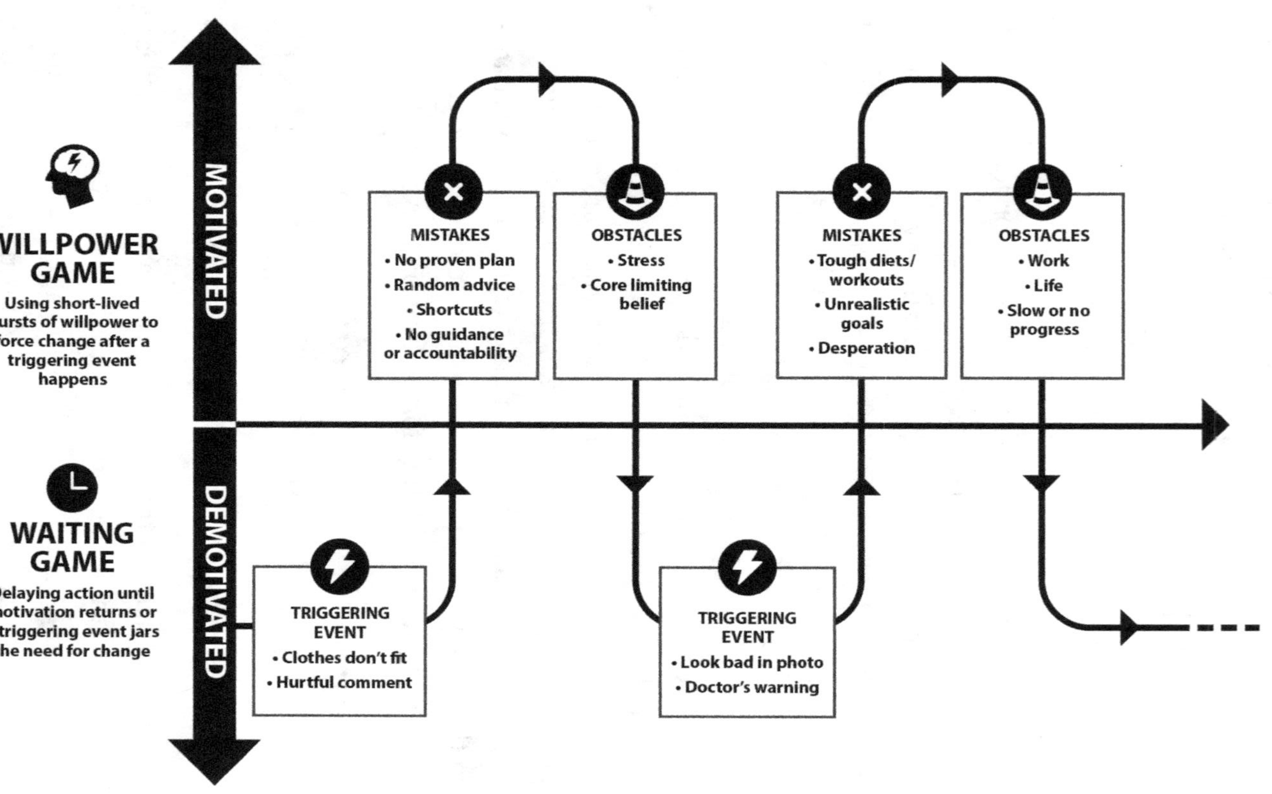

WILLPOWER GAME
Using short-lived bursts of willpower to force change after a triggering event happens
WAITING GAME
Delaying action until motivation returns or a triggering event jars the need for change
MOTIVATED
DEMOTIVATED
TRIGGERING EVENT
• Clothes don't fit
• Hurtful comment
MISTAKES
• No proven plan
• Random advice
• Shortcuts
• No guidance or accountability
OBSTACLES
• Stress
• Core limiting belief
TRIGGERING EVENT
• Look bad in photo
• Doctor's warning
MISTAKES
• Tough diets/ workouts
• Unrealistic goals
• Desperation
OBSTACLES
• Work
• Life
• Slow or no progress

This pattern is not uncommon. My client Eric would struggle with this pattern. He would start out on his fitness goals feeling "like gangbusters," as he'd say, until something would come up and knock him off his rhythm. A bad day would turn into a bad week. A bad week into a bad month. Inevitably, his motivation would wane until he'd throw in the proverbial towel and find himself back at square one. (Sound familiar?)

Needless to say, the ability to stay motivated consistently is vital to maintaining our results. So, it's essential we transform our relationship with motivation if we're going to attain, and maintain, our body and health where we want them.

We also have to make sure that we're not making other mistakes that can hurt our motivation, like buying into myths.

PEOPLE BELIEVE MOTIVATION MYTHS THAT CAN CAUSE MISTAKES

If we don't understand motivation correctly, we can't fully harness its power. Understanding the reality of motivation helps you avoid the pitfalls of common myths when it comes to ensuring you maintain your body transformation.

So let's get clear on what motivation is and isn't.

MYTH #1: MOTIVATION IS REQUIRED TO GET INTO ACTION

How often have you felt this way? You are feeling bad about not having made much progress in your body goals lately, so your motivation is in the toilet. Because your motivation is in the toilet, you numb out with food or social media, and don't do anything to make a change. Then, the next day, you feel bad again, so you numb out again. You are now officially in the Cycle of Stuck.

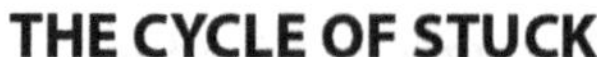

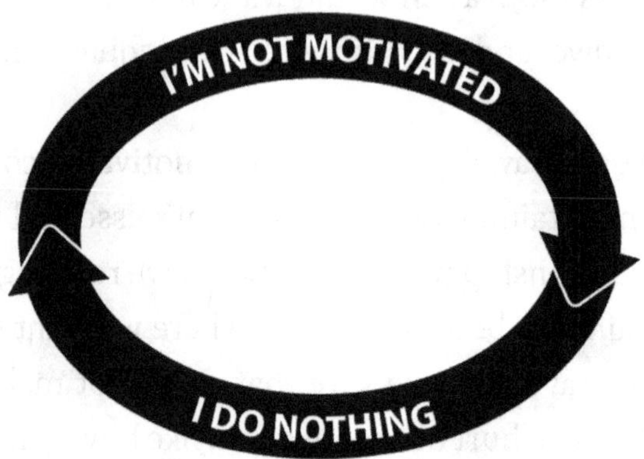

To say the least, being stuck in the cycle of stuck . . . sucks. (Say that ten times fast!)

Unfortunately, most people get stuck in this pattern. That's because taking action without feeling motivated is a skill most people haven't developed.

If they're not motivated, they don't get in action, and that's that. No motivation, no action. Just waiting. I've seen people settle for operating this way for weeks, months or even years.

Waiting around for motivation to suddenly fall out of the sky or for the mailman to deliver it is not a winning strategy.

Reality: Action Comes Before Motivation

Contrary to popular opinion, motivation is NOT required in order to take action. In fact, motivation does NOT come before action. It's the other way around: action comes ***before*** motivation.

In the book, *The Motivation Myth*, author Jeff Haden states, "You feel motivated because you took action. Motivation is a result, not a pre-condition. You don't need motivation to break a sweat. Break a sweat, and you'll feel motivated."[17]

Our brains are wired to move towards pleasure. If you take action towards something that will give you pleasure or be beneficial, you start to feel good. That good feeling is your brain rewarding you for taking action with a small hit of dopamine, a feel good hormone. This good feeling, in turn, makes you want to do more of that action. This is the mechanism for how new habits start. Taking that action brings forth the motivation needed to continue.

Doctor of Psychology Emily Guarnotta says, "When you do something enjoyable . . . your brain releases dopamine, causing you to feel good. The brain then remembers how this experience is rewarding and seeks it out again . . . dopamine is responsible for us repeating behaviors or activities that are pleasurable."[18]

The goal then, is to take action—even when we don't feel motivated—so we can keep our motivation going, instead of waiting for it to find us.

MYTH #2: MOTIVATION IS A FEELING OF EXCITEMENT OR DESIRE

Excitement runs high when we commit to a new goal or endeavor such as starting a business, entering a new relationship, or changing our bodies. This initial feeling is great; it means the goal is important to us. But excitement eventually fades, especially when things get challenging. *(Ask any couple that's been together for more than a year and you'll see what I mean!)* If you depend on feeling excited to get motivated enough to take action consistently, your progress is sure to grind to a halt as soon as the excitement of pursuing your body transformation goal fizzles out.

Reality: Seeing Progress Keeps You Motivated

Seeing progress is better than excitement. We talked about how taking action towards important goals gives us a little feel-good dopamine hit. If the action you take makes actual progress toward the goal, you get an even bigger dopamine hit. Our brains reward us when we make progress because we're biased toward growth. As author William S. Burroughs says, "When you stop growing, you start dying."

In this sense, humans are like plants—we're either flourishing or slowly withering away. If you do something that helps you to grow or progress, you're in alignment with your nature as a person. This will feel good and make you want to do more of it. The opposite is also true. If our actions don't lead to progress, we'll get frustrated and demotivated.

This concept builds on the first one that says we must take action in order to feel motivated. When the actions we take make some kind of progress toward our goal, it compounds the "feel good" effect. This combination of taking action and seeing progress is very powerful for both staying motivated and sustaining habits. This takes us out of the cycle of stuck and puts us in what I call "The Motivation Loop."

MOTIVATION LOOP

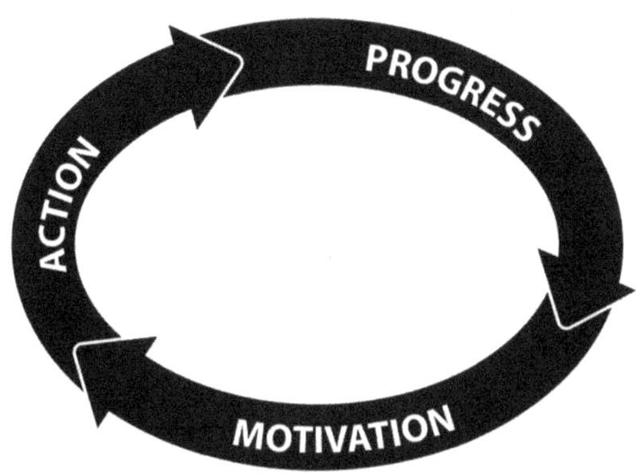

MYTH #3: MOTIVATION IS ABOUT GETTING "PUMPED UP"

Sure, watching or hearing something motivational can give us a temporary injection of motivation. There's certainly no shortage of gurus and influencers waiting to pump us up, yell at us, call us out for making excuses, or aggressively push us to "stop being so soft." But true motivation is not about pumping up or shaming people. Techniques such as these are temporary at best and overbearing at worst. But feel free to judge for yourself.

Have you ever seen or read some content that was trying to pump you up?

Did you stay motivated?

Did you change your behavior long-term?

(Didn't think so.)

While that type of content might get you temporarily excited, that feeling is fleeting (see myth #2 above). Once it fades, you're back to facing the same gravitational pull of de-motivation.

Reality: Support Structures Will Keep You on Track

When the pump-up guru's rant is long forgotten, you can turn to something that's longer lasting to keep you on track and motivated: the structures you put in place. Setting up things like an accountability partner, clear goals with consequences, and a physical environment that ensures success (for example, keeping tempting junk food out of sight) will go a long way towards keeping you motivated and ensuring you see progress.

MYTH #4: MOTIVATION COMES FROM WILLPOWER

As mentioned, many people try to rely on their personal willpower to get to their goal—they just grit their teeth and gut it out. They'll endure miserable diets or do tons of exercises they don't enjoy, usually because of a goal set out of desperation, like, "I need a hot bod to stick it to my ex to show them what they lost out on!" For most mortals, willpower only lasts for a few weeks. After that, the person revolts against the diet or program and ends up going the other extreme of binging on comfort foods or stopping their exercise completely. Going from one extreme to another like this is not exactly the best way to find balance, nor is it good for your metabolism.

Reality: Inspiration Is an Endless Source of Motivation

Instead of relying on willpower there's a more potent and infinite source of motivation you can tap into: inspiration. By aligning your thoughts with what inspires you, you will have an endless source of inspiration waiting to "pull" you towards your goal. Conversely, willpower requires you to "push" and force your way to the goal. What do you think is more effortless? Being pulled towards your goal, or having to push your way to it?

From a metaphysical view, when we are inspired we are connected to our true essence. We're accessing source energy and the deeper wisdom of the universe. Unlike willpower, source energy is infinite.

THERE'S HOPE FOR WAVERING MOTIVATION

The inertia from having completely lost your motivation not only feels lousy, it takes a lot of effort to overcome. In a sense, motivation works kind of like a plane. It takes a lot more jet fuel for a plane to take off from the ground than to keep it flying once it's reached altitude. Similarly, it takes a lot more willpower to climb out of the cycle of stuck and get motivated than it does to keep your motivation going once it's already high.

So the approach we want to take is, instead of letting motivation go all the way down, and then having to drum up massive effort to get it back up again, we want to keep your motivation at cruising altitude (with small, consistent actions and progress) and never let it get too low. Once it's up there, it will be easy to sustain without a lot of focus, effort, or willpower.

If motivation has caused you to struggle in the past, know that help is on the way. In Chapter 17, "Shift #3: Activate Your Motivators" you will learn some powerful mindset techniques for keeping your motivation high consistently.

For now, try out this quick action to give your motivation level a kick in the pants.

QUICK ACTION

We learned that motivation comes from taking action and getting results. When we keep our promises to ourselves, we feel better and our motivation continues to grow and grow. So this week, make a small promise to yourself that you know you can easily keep.

If you've been sedentary, commit to going for a post-dinner walk. Just one twenty minute stroll. If you've been somewhat active, make it a brisk 20-minute walk. Set a timer for ten minutes and walk away from your home or office, then when it goes off, walk the same way back. Ten minutes out, ten minutes back. Don't worry about getting geared up. You can just take your walk in your regular clothes.

Just make and keep this promise to yourself, and get those steps in. Taking the action will make you feel good, and put you right back into the Motivation Loop!

50-YEAR OLD FURNITURE EXEC KICKS BAD HABITS, A TOXIC RELATIONSHIP, AND IS "FLOORED" BY HIS RESULTS

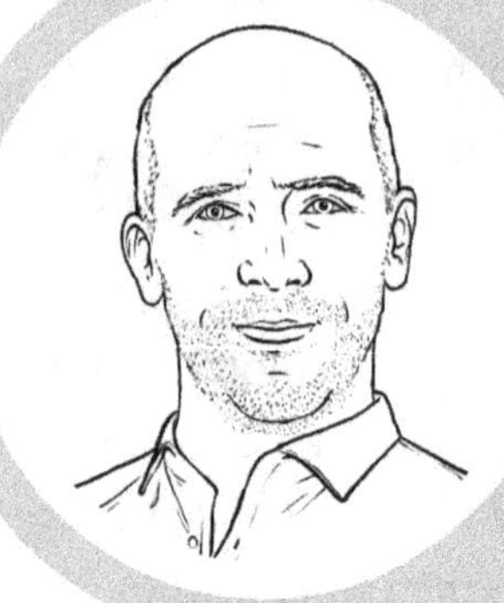

I used to feel tired and unmotivated all the time. But you helped me get back on the ball and showed me how to eat the right way. Without you, I'd still be struggling. Thank you! –Steve

THE SITUATION

Steve was fast approaching his 50th birthday and wanted to turn things around in terms of his body, health, and confidence. He was dealing with several toxic relationships (ex-girlfriend, mother) in his personal life and to cope with the heavy toll they were taking on his emotions he would smoke marijuana. Getting high would inevitably lead to junk food cravings. Over time, these munchies caused weight gain and gut dysbiosis.

Steve's energy levels were also down, and he would tire quickly. Afternoon crashes were the norm. He would eat haphazardly, eating out daily and grabbing whatever was available to get him through the day. His confidence was down, he rarely kept good habits, and he was no longer as socially active as in the past. It was time for a change.

THE SOLUTION

With his permission, we coached Steve on how to create more workable situations with the toxic relationships he was in by bravely speaking up and setting boundaries. We guided him on making better choices when eating out while helping him adopt more weekly meal planning and prepping to take back control over what goes into his body. We also custom-tailored a minimalist exercise routine that helped Steve get an effective minimum dose of activity on weeks he worked long hours or had to travel to client sites to supervise furniture installs.

THE TRANSFORMATION

"Before, I didn't have the knowledge of what or how to eat. I would exercise but it wasn't working. I used to feel tired and unmotivated all the time. But you helped me get back on the ball and showed me how to eat the right way. Without you, I'd still be struggling. Thank you!"

Through our work with Steve, he gained greater clarity around how, when, and what to eat, and he exercised more than he had in many years. He was able to lose over thirty pounds and improve his digestion issues while dramatically reducing his visceral fat levels. He tactfully created a healthy distance among the people in his personal life who were draining him, making him more calm, less stressed, and much happier. As a result his junk food binges went way down as Steve reduced his reliances on marijuana.

Best of all, Steve went to Las Vegas to celebrate his 50th birthday and felt proud of himself. He said he never imagined making the type of progress he made in his body during his transformation program.

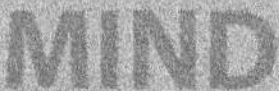

Emotional Eating
Limiting Beliefs
Wavering Motivation

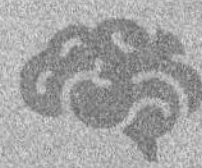

BODY

Slowing Metabolism

CHAPTER 7

CHALLENGE #4: Slowing Metabolism

"You're never too old for anything!"
—Betty White

OK, we just covered the three main challenges our mind creates that makes it hard to keep our bodies how we want them (emotional eating, limiting beliefs, and wavering motivation). Now, let's look at how our body creates challenges, especially as we age.

Let's face it. You and I are not spring chickens anymore.

At this stage of the game, our bodies are not what they used to be in our younger years.

There was a time when we had a well-oiled metabolism, finely tuned hormones, shiny joints, and the freedom to run with the wind.

Now that we're in midlife, those days are long gone.

In turn, we have to get smarter and more strategic about how we solve the challenges that this stage of life brings if we want to keep our bodies healthy and fit well into our later years.

Being over forty usually means added stress from the increased responsibilities of work and family, and it also brings us a body that (sadly) is starting to go downhill. Factors such as metabolic decline, changing hormones, greater potential for injuries, and the impact of medications are some of the main reasons this stage of life can make it harder for us to achieve the body, health, and energy we seek.

One of the biggest challenges of this stage of life is a slowing metabolism.

Around the age of forty, many people experience a decrease in their metabolic rate. It gradually slows until we're about sixty years old and then slows at a faster rate from there. [19]

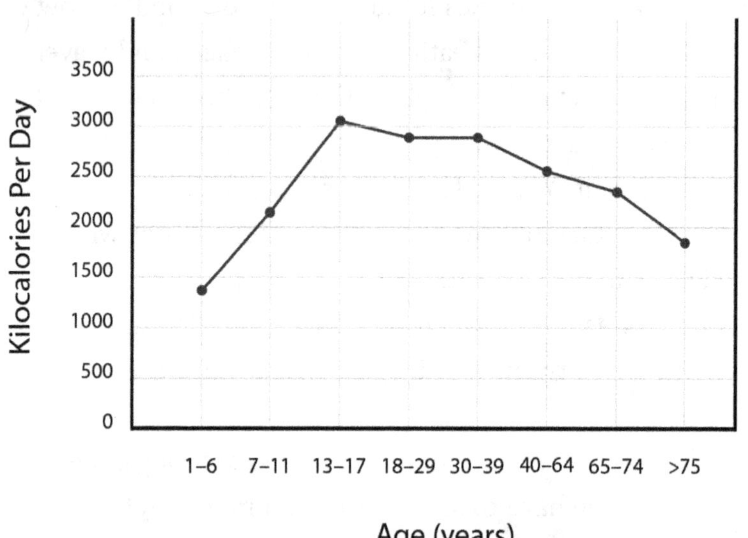

The reasons for this are both physiological as well as lifestyle related.

From a physiological standpoint, men experience a slow and steady metabolic decline caused primarily by sarcopenia (muscle loss). This is caused by declining testosterone levels, which dip by about 1% every year after a man reaches thirty.

For women, however, metabolic decline can happen more acutely due to menopause. This transition results in a variety of changes, chief among them a significant reduction of her reproductive hormones, including estrogen and progesterone.[20]

These hormonal changes can trigger physiological symptoms such as hot flashes. As her reproductive hormones diminish, it can give way to other hormonal changes that actually make it harder to lose body fat and easier to gain it.

First, some women may experience a rise in insulin levels, which can make it harder for the body to burn stored fat. That's because insulin production by the pancreas shuts off the hormone glucagon, one of our main mobilizers of stored fat.

The second menopause-related change that can make it harder for some women to lose body fat is an increase in cortisol levels. As I will cover shortly, chronically elevated cortisol levels can lead to fat gain due to increases in blood sugar levels and a slowing of the metabolism.

Both sexes also experience metabolic decline due to lifestyle factors that can impact the metabolism. This includes enduring higher stress levels, being more sedentary, getting suboptimal sleep, and using medications that impact their hormones and metabolism.

CAN THIS BE DONE AT ANY AGE?

For now, know that reversing metabolic decline is totally possible to do, at any age.

How old is too old?

There really isn't an age limit on the body's ability to transform.

Our miraculous bodies are designed to function well into our final days on this planet. Whether it's healing from a cut, digesting food, or adding muscle, these functions are already pre-programmed, as long as we treat our body the way it's meant to be treated.

Does it get harder when we age?

Sure.

But that doesn't mean we are no longer able to do it.

You already saw how my client, Eric, the former airline executive, was able to attain a six-pack at the age of sixty-five.

My client, Jill, a 55-year old IT executive, had this to say:

"Deekron, it's really amazing, my metabolism has reset. When I'm good and follow your plan I lose weight. But when I'm bad, I don't gain any weight! You guys jumped started my metabolism!"—Jill

But first she had to overcome some struggles. You'll hear her story shortly.

Needless to say, a slower metabolism leads to fewer calories burned per day. This makes it easier to store, and harder to lose, body fat.

It also leads to decreased energy levels.

THERE'S HOPE FOR A SLOWING METABOLISM

One of the key strategies we employ to help elevate an over-40 metabolism is through strength training workouts. There are three primary ways strength training aids in boosting the metabolism.

First, when we strength train, we build lean muscle, which elevates your resting metabolism rate.[21] Second, as a form of exercise, a strength training session demands energy and thus, burns calories. A proper strength training workout can burn up to 200 calories per 30-minute bout.[22]

Third, and most impactful, is the fact that strength training is the best modality to trigger what's known as "the afterburn effect." By causing metabolic stress, a proper strength training workout can keep your metabolism elevated for hours after your workout is over, burning "bonus" calories. (Pretty cool, right? You'll learn more about how to do this soon.)

When you use the right strength training strategy, ***and*** provide your body with optimal nutrition and sleep to support your training efforts (as well as your busy day) you'll take advantage of these mechanisms above to elevate your metabolism and keep it high as you age. This is exactly what you're going to learn how to do in Part III of this book, so keep going!

QUICK ACTION

Remember that elevating your metabolism the right way requires adding muscle tone by aligning your training, eating, and recovery towards this goal. Do one thing this week that will move you forward in at least one of those three areas.

Thought starters: do some body weight exercises (that are appropriate for your level); you can find some on YouTube. Eat in a way that supports a faster metabolism; elevating your protein intake is a great place to start. Improve your sleep by not using devices in your bedroom.

In Chapter 19, "Shift #4: Train for Strength" I will be going over strategies to optimize your strength training to get maximum metabolic benefits. You will also find a Strength Training Action Plan you can do at home with minimal equipment. For now, let's cover another body-related challenge that makes it harder for professionals over-40 to achieve their desired body and health: changing hormones.

CHALLENGE #4: SLOWING METABOLISM

JILL, A 55-YEAR-OLD IT EXECUTIVE REPROGRAMS HER METABOLISM IN HER MID-50'S

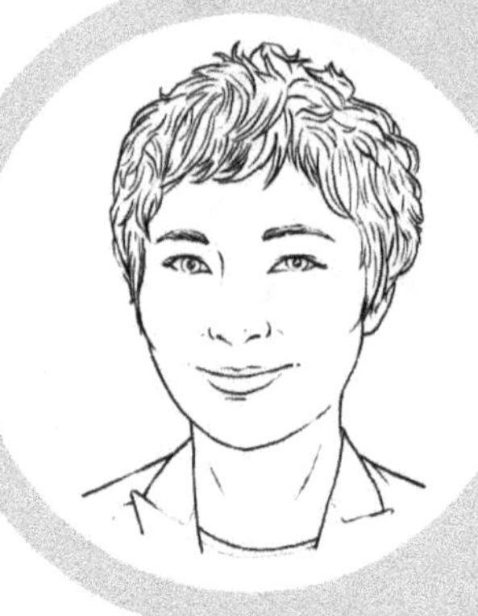

All my confusion went away when I started following *The Nine Shifts*.
–Jill

THE SITUATION

Jill had gone through menopause, which had slowed her metabolism and led to her gaining body fat, primarily in her love handles. While she had tried numerous ways to get the fat off, including walking and online Zumba classes, she saw little result. She was left frustrated and unsure about what to do, especially at her age. Jill wanted to get her body fat down and overcome the challenges posed by working from home and sitting all day in front of a computer.

THE SOLUTION

We helped Jill align her training, nutrition, and recovery to add more muscle tone in order to elevate her metabolism. From a mindset perspective, we coached Jill to overcome her (common) fear that eating more would result in her gaining weight and we taught her how to strategically eat more. This allowed Jill to properly nourish her body and support the energy demands of her metabolism-boosting workouts, as well as her grueling work schedule. We crafted a training plan that could be done from home in a flexible, doable, and enjoyable way. Jill confessed that even though she "absolutely hated" doing all of the different squats we had prescribed in her plan, she loved the results they were getting her!

THE TRANSFORMATION

As a result of us helping Jill elevate her metabolism, she lost close to 25 lb in her first three months and completely melted away her stubborn love handles. She was pleasantly surprised that she was able to accomplish this at her age. Jill was also happy to have a clear routine and lifestyle she could follow and not let working from home and sitting all day doing IT work impede her from achieving a body she's now very proud of.

Jill used to have a lot of confusion around losing weight and how to transform her body, and now she says, "All my confusion went away when I went through your program."

Emotional Eating
Limiting Beliefs
Wavering Motivation

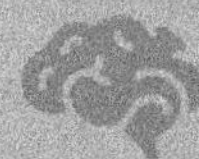

BODY

Slowing Metabolism
Changing Hormones

CHAPTER 8

CHALLENGE #5: Changing Hormones

"Hormones get no respect. We think of them as the elusive chemicals that make us a bit moody, but these magical little molecules do so much more."
—Susannah Cahalan

As we reach mid-life, not only does our metabolism slow, our hormones begin to change. Like with our metabolism, aging and lifestyle choices impact our hormonal levels in ways that can make it harder to attain and maintain the body and quality of life we seek.

In this chapter, we will briefly touch on the hormones that are key to our body transformation goals, including insulin, cortisol, and our reproductive hormones. We will close out the chapter by touching on the subject of gut health, an often overlooked area that is connected to our hormonal system and is essential to our well being and body transformation goals.

THE ROLE OF HORMONES IN THE BODY

As chemical messengers that regulate different functions in our body, hormones manage many of the body's key processes. They play a key role in the functioning of our blood pressure, appetite, mood, sleep, libido, reproduction, cell growth, body temperature, energy, and (most importantly for our purposes), the metabolism.

When our hormones are working properly we feel good, have lots of energy, a good appetite, sleep well, handle stress well, and we keep our weight in a healthy range. When our hormones are not working properly, life can be more challenging. We can become more irritable, depressed, sluggish, experience sleep issues, and gain weight.

The mind and the body have a self-referential relationship. To ensure homeostasis and that everything stays in balance, the brain and the body are always working together via what's known as a "negative feedback loop." Based on the feedback it's getting about the body, the hypothalamus will act like a regulator (similar to a thermostat), turning on or turning off the production of different hormones based on what it's sensing in the body. For example, if you haven't eaten in a while, and the brain senses that blood sugar is dropping, it will increase your hunger hormone, ghrelin, which will make you feel hungry and prompt you to seek out food.

HORMONAL IMBALANCES (AND DISRUPTORS)

Generally speaking, an imbalance in our hormones occurs when there is either too much or too little presence of that hormone in the body. Some of the common causes of hormonal imbalances include:

- **Poor nutrition**—Highly processed foods and refined carbs can cause inflammation and disrupt key hormones such as insulin, which can lead to insulin resistance and Type 2 Diabetes.
- **Malnutrition**—Lack of key, hormone-dependent nutrients such as Vitamin D or Zinc (among others) can affect hormone levels.
- **Obesity**—Being obese can disrupt key hormones in the body, including elevating estrogen levels and suppressing human growth hormone.
- **Life stage**—At mid-life, a man's testosterone levels begin to decline, while a female who goes through menopause will emerge with diminished sex hormones, and the possibility of elevated insulin and cortisol levels.
- **Diseases**—An autoimmune disease such as Hashimoto's Thyroiditis attacks the thyroid gland and disrupts its ability to produce enough of the thyroid hormone T4, leading to an underactive thyroid and a slower metabolism.
- **Environmental disruptors**—Chemicals and toxins known as endocrine-disrupting chemicals (EDCs) found in the environment, including drinking water, the air, plastic packaging, household cleaners, and personal care products have been shown to affect hormonal levels, including impairing sex hormones and fertility.

- **Medications**—Certain pharmaceutical medications can impact hormones in the body; antidepressants have been shown to disrupt thyroid function, growth hormone, estrogen and testosterone.

On this last point, since 66% of U.S. adults take at least one type of pharmaceutical drug, it's important for us to account for the impact of medications on the body and health of the typical over-40 professional.[23]

THE IMPACT OF HORMONAL IMBALANCES

An imbalance or suboptimal state in our hormone levels can lead to a slowing of metabolic function and impairment of other important functions. This situation can make it harder to keep our body, health, and performance where we want them to be.

The list of possible hormonal disruptions and their impact on our bodies is long and complex. For expediency, let's briefly cover the more common hormonal challenges that most people face (and that you may encounter as well). These are the ones I see most often in my practice:

- insulin resistance (high blood sugar)
- low testosterone
- hypothyroidism and Hashimoto's thyroiditis
- adrenal fatigue
- menopause-related hormonal changes

INSULIN RESISTANCE (HIGH BLOOD SUGAR)

Insulin is a storage hormone secreted by the pancreas and is required to transport the nutrients that we consume like carbs, protein, and fats into our cells. When the body becomes less sensitive to the hormone insulin, a condition known as insulin resistance (IR) results. Having IR makes it harder for insulin to clear glucose from the bloodstream. This results in less sugar being stored in our muscles, liver, and other cells (where it belongs), and more of it floating around in the blood and being deposited in our fat cells.

This adds to stored body fat levels and increases the number of fat molecules in the bloodstream, known as our triglycerides. This can lead to a hardening of arteries, which increases the risk of a stroke, heart attack, or heart disease.[24]

If it goes on for long enough, IR can create a cluster of risk factors for the heart, a condition known as metabolic syndrome. This is when the person suffers simultaneously from obesity, high blood pressure, elevated fasting glucose, high triglyceride levels, and low HDL (good) cholesterol levels.[25]

What's more, constantly elevated blood sugar levels due to IR prevent the body from using stored body fat for energy, making it harder to lose weight. Worse still, consistently high blood sugar, if left unchecked (i.e., many months or years), can result in damage to our nerves, blood vessels, kidneys, eyes, heart, brain, digestive tract, and other organs. This can lead to many deleterious health outcomes like obesity, heart disease, neuropathy, Alzheimer's, organ failure and, at the extreme, the potential for amputation of limbs. (Scary, I know.)

Sadly, IR has been on the rise. Thanks to the standard American diet and the plethora of unhealthy, processed foods in our food supply, supermarkets, and restaurants, a full 40% of Americans have developed insulin resistance.[26]

Even if someone doesn't have high blood sugar or insulin resistance currently, the potential to develop it increases with age.

This means we have to prevent it from ever developing, even if we're healthy now, or we may risk significant consequences to our health in the future. If we have already developed it, we must be diligent to reverse it immediately.

The good news (yes there is good news) is that IR is reversible. It can be reversed, but ***only*** by consistently following the right habits around nutrition, exercise, sleep, and stress management—everything you are learning about in this book.

Using our *Nine Shifts* methodology and empathetic coaching, my team and I have helped numerous clients bring down blood sugar levels—greatly improving their A1C—including those who came to us with a prediabetes or Type 2 diabetes diagnosis.

LOW TESTOSTERONE (LOW T)

Low testosterone levels can affect both men and women, but because it's the primary male sex hormone, it affects males more.

Testosterone is a man's mojo. It controls his mood, keeps muscle mass on his frame, keeps him strong, sexually active, keeps energy and stamina high, keeps his mood positive. When it's low, life can really suck for him. He's lethargic and loses interest in things. Worse, it keeps his metabolism slow and body fat high.

Sorry to say, but the news for us fellas isn't very good. As mentioned, men begin to lose 1% of their testosterone (T) every year starting around the age of thirty. By the time a man is fifty, his T is roughly 40% (less than half) of what it was in his twenties.[27] Sadly, T levels have been decreasing in men overall. An age-independent study showed that testosterone levels have dropped by 25% in men over the last two decades, an alarming trend for men's health.[28]

When I work with male clients one of my main goals is to ensure that we're keeping his T levels high. I'm happy to say that I helped my client Chris, a high-powered NYC attorney (who you will "meet" soon) boost his T levels by over 50%, naturally; no drugs or testosterone replacement therapy needed.

Sometimes, medicinal approaches such as testosterone replacement therapy (TRT/HRT) may be necessary. In these cases, we have our clients consult with our functional medicine practitioners and our partner clinics to help regulate any hormonal deficiencies.

HYPOTHYROIDISM AND HASHIMOTO'S THYROIDITIS

Hypothyroidism occurs when the body's thyroid gland underproduces thyroid hormones due to factors such as nutritional deficiencies or high stress. In the case of Hashimoto's thyroiditis, which is an autoimmune disease, the body confuses a thyroid hormone with an intruder and the immune system begins to attack the thyroid gland, causing an underproduction of the hormone T4, which impairs thyroid function.[29]

As the main regulator of how much energy we burn, our thyroid underperforming can result in reduced energy and weight gain. Hypothyroidism is more common in females and can sometimes begin after menopause. With hypothyroidism, it's important to address any nutritional deficiencies or inflammatory responses that can make the condition worse. A proper supplementation plan, along with stress management, and appropriate exercise can help overcome hypothyroidism.

Two of my female clients featured in this book Deborah, the real estate agency owner, and Tammy, the senior SaaS sales executive, both have Hashimoto's. So does Walter, a military vet that you'll meet soon. I'm happy to say that with our *Nine Shifts* method and coaching (combined with their ongoing medicinal treatment for their condition) they were able to have great success in transforming their bodies in spite of their thyroid disease.

ADRENAL FATIGUE

Our adrenal glands sit on top of our kidneys and are responsible for secreting several key hormones including cortisol, one of our primary energy mobilizers.

Adrenal fatigue can be caused by extended periods of high stress, or by autoimmune diseases such as Epstein-Barr syndrome. When our adrenals malfunction, they impair the body's ability to produce cortisol and generate energy when it's needed. This can make it difficult to do even basic tasks like walk, get dressed, or even get out of bed.

Besides energy mismanagement, adrenal fatigue can result in weight gain. Because adrenal fatigue is not an officially recognized condition by western medicine, there are no pharmaceutical drugs designed to treat it. Treatment usually involves natural supplementation to improve adrenal function and manage cortisol levels. Sufferers of adrenal fatigue must also make changes in their lifestyle to reduce stress from all sources, including emotional, physical, and external.

MENOPAUSE

When a female reaches midlife, her body starts winding down her reproductive system. This transition known as menopause, is marked by significant hormonal changes in her body.

Key female hormones needed for fertility, such as estrogen and progesterone, are significantly reduced. Simultaneously, cortisol and insulin may become elevated in some women. Not only do these hormonal changes come with potential symptoms like hot flashes, night sweats, and emotional swings but it may also impact body composition. As cortisol goes up, her body can become more sensitive to stress, leading to some of the cortisol-driven reactions in the body like elevated sugar levels, a slowing metabolism, cravings for comfort foods, and potential for muscle loss.

As insulin levels rise, the potential for developing insulin resistance increases and maintaining her desired weight can become more difficult. In fact, some women that go through menopause can end up gaining weight and may even get diagnosed with prediabetes or even Type 2 diabetes.

With the right approach, menopause does not have to be an insurmountable obstacle for a woman who is trying to keep her body optimal. In fact, almost every one of the women featured in this book had gone through menopause before they started working with us. It's very possible for a woman to transform her body post-menopause. My client Tammy is living proof; you'll read about her transformation journey shortly.

GUT HEALTH AND DIGESTIVE ISSUES

The gut refers to our gastrointestinal system. It includes the esophagus, stomach, and small and large intestines. Our gut is responsible for digestion, processing, and absorption of the foods we eat.

Living inside our gut is the microbiome, an ecosystem of bacteria that plays a key role in digestion and metabolism. A truly astonishing organ, it weighs approximately 2.5 lb and is estimated to contain between 39 trillion and 100 trillion microbial cells that play a key role in digestion as well as immunity.

There's a tight connection between the brain and the gut, which are linked via what is called the vagus nerve, the longest running nerve in the body. The vagus nerve acts as a central monitoring station, constantly communicating between the brain and our main organs.

Because the gut plays such a critical role in processing food into energy and nutrients that our cells need to function, maintaining our gut health in an optimal state is essential to having the health, body, and energy we seek.

GUT HEALTH DISRUPTORS

Hormonal imbalances, including the ones mentioned above, such as hypothyroidism and insulin resistance, can affect our gut health and digestion. Additionally, when one has dysbiosis, an imbalance in the gastrointestinal tract, such as Small Intestinal Bacterial Overgrowth (SIBO), Irritable Bowel Syndrome (IBS), leaky gut (intestinal permeability) or infections like candida or H. Pylori, this will also create gut health and digestive issues.

When our gut health gets disrupted, the main issues that arise are malnutrition, inflammation, and digestive discomfort.

Some of the leading sources of gut disruption include:

- excessive alcohol consumption
- long-term use of pharmaceutical medication
- extended periods of intense stress
- overconsumption of inflammatory foods, especially refined sugars
- food allergies and sensitivities
- prolonged bouts of constipation
- autoimmune diseases that affect the gut
- injury to the digestive tract

Because professionals over the age of forty deal with several of the items on this list it's important to account for their impact on our gut if the goal is to be optimal in body and health.

THERE'S HOPE FOR CHANGING HORMONES

As you can see, both our hormones and our digestive system play key roles in keeping us healthy, functioning well, staying lean, and feeling our best. It should also be obvious that there are many factors that can influence our hormonal profile and our gut health. But by limiting the hormonal and gut health disruptors you just learned about, you can limit the challenges they can pose to your body transformation goals.

QUICK ACTION

Having quality nutrition—eating enough calories and getting proper nutrients—plays a primary role in keeping your hormones and your gut health happy. Conversely, processed foods that cause inflammation can hurt your hormonal profile and disrupt the gut.

Reflect on what processed or inflammatory foods you might be having. Common examples include refined carbs and sugar/sugary items, gluten, soybeans or soybean oil, corn-based products (like fried chips or corn syrup), and alcohol. Identify one that you have most often that you can live without, and seek to reduce it gradually.

Your hormones and your gut will thank you!

FINANCE EXECUTIVE DUMPS THE EXTRA WORKLOAD FOR A BETTER BOTTOM LINE

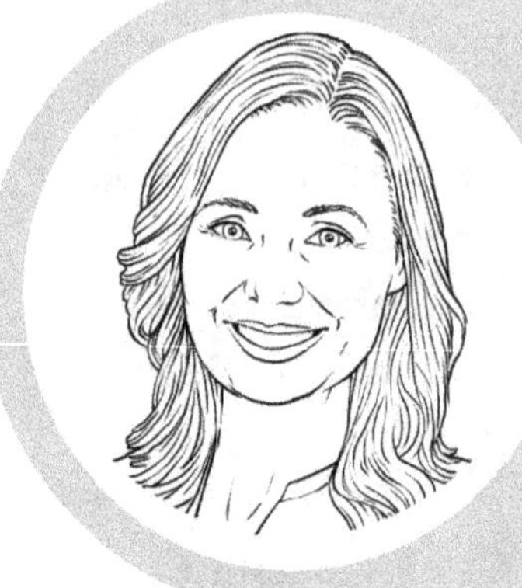

There's a synergy to this program. It all works together. It's everything you need to get you to your goal.

–Tammy

THE SITUATION

When Tammy hit menopause, she experienced hormonal changes and a slowing metabolism. This, combined with the stress of dealing with her mom's end-of-life situation, and taking anti-anxiety medication, led to a perfect storm of health decline. She gained 70 lb, mostly in her midsection, and her A1C shot up, which resulted in a prediabetes diagnosis. She lamented that she felt very "heavy" in her body. Her energy levels had tanked. Basic activities like climbing stairs or chasing after her nephew had become difficult, leaving her extremely frustrated. Additionally, Tammy really hated how she now looked in photos.

Because Tammy had been thin her whole life up to this point, having to lose weight was unchartered territory for her. "How am I going to do this, at my age, no less?" she bemoaned.

Tammy didn't know where, or how, to start. She was left feeling demotivated and stuck.

THE SOLUTION

We first worked with Tammy on her mindset and her motivation levels. By making it easy for her to get started and get some easy wins under her belt to build momentum, we gave her the jumpstart she needed. We also coached her on how to set boundaries at work because the departure of a coworker resulted in Tammy's workload doubling and the constant overtime was causing Tammy to miss her workouts every week. (Yes, she's a people pleaser.)

Reviewing Tammy's lab results, we gave her nutrition, lifestyle, and supplementation recommendations to keep her blood sugar under control. Giving Tammy a very flexible meal plan that allowed her to eat pretty much anything she wanted, as long as the sources were clean and she hit her macronutrient (protein, fat, and carb) targets, made it a sustainable approach for her to maintain consistently.

THE TRANSFORMATION

Tammy was able to lose close to 30 lb and reduce her menopause belly significantly. She felt much lighter in her body and had a lot more energy.

Tammy quickly graduated from working in her basement with resistance bands to feeling confident enough to go start training at her local gym again. She felt like she was in a better groove with her habits and was clear on what to do each week to continue the momentum she had built.

Tammy credits the comprehensive nature of the program as a key to her success. She loved the age-appropriate nature of the workouts, flexibility in meals, adaptability to her schedule, and our ongoing support around mindset and bloodwork. "There's a synergy to this program. It all works together. It's everything you need to get you to your goal."

MIND
Emotional Eating
Limiting Beliefs
Wavering Motivation

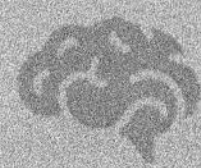

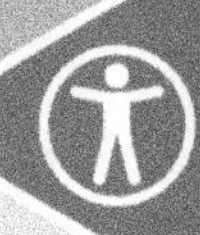

BODY
Slowing Metabolism
Changing Hormones
Injuries & Limitations

CHAPTER 9

CHALLENGE #6: Injuries & Limitations

"An injury is much sooner forgotten than an insult."
—Philip Stanhope

Most over-40 professionals that I know are driven and competitive in nature. We don't just want to be our best, we want to be ***the best***. Your competitiveness may have driven you to play sports when you were younger. You may still be playing sports now (or not).

Either way, I salute you.

As the son of a former pro athlete (my dad played rugby professionally in Romania), I played almost every sport growing up thanks to his encouragement. I believe that the way playing sports develops our bodies, character, social skills, and self-expression is second to none for personal growth. Plus, it can be super fun—especially when we win, right?!

If you played sports when you were younger or still participate today, your body has probably been through some beatings. Even if you didn't play sports very much throughout your life, the fact remains that our bodies are aging by the day. Frailer bones, creakier joints, excess body fat, and tight muscles from sitting all day predispose us to potential injuries. Take a look at the most common emergency department visits in the U.S.[30]

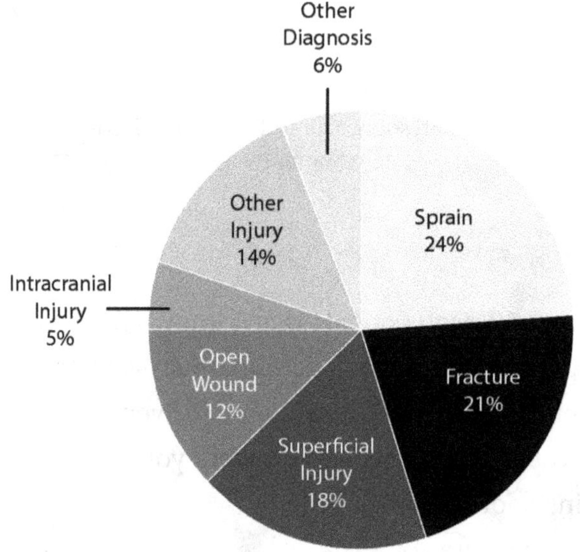

That's why the exercise regimen you follow has to be age and ability appropriate.

Needless to say, most of the flashy, intense workouts that the 20-somethings do on Instagram to get clicks will most likely throw your back out faster than you can say "BENGAY."

Perhaps you've had injuries or operations in the past. Maybe you have some nagging injuries that bother you today. Whatever the case, staying active (and lean) over the long run means being able to work around current limitations and preventing injuries as we age.

I WANT TO HELP YOU STAY ACTIVE FOR LIFE

Thanks to a lifetime of being athletic, I've had more injuries than I care to recount. Name the joint or body part, and I've hurt it at some point. I've been through almost every therapy you can imagine; cortisone shots, deep tissue massage, physical therapy, sports massage, acupuncture, reiki, occlusion bands, needling, PRP injections, peptide injections, and even surgery.

You get the idea. A lifetime of playing sports, skiing moguls, running endurance races like marathons, and lifting iron since the age of thirteen has resulted in a beating on this body. Now that I'm in my fifties, I have to be super smart and careful with how I train because I plan on doing this for many more years to come.

And I'd like to empower you to do the same.

In fact, I made it a point to get certified in Pain-Free Performance (I'm a PPSC certified coach) so I can properly program age-and-ability-appropriate workouts for my over-40 clientele that bulletproof their bodies.

This way, you can enjoy a lifetime of pain-free strength and do the activities of your choosing, for as long as you choose to do them.

Here's a pretty important change you have to make in your approach if you plan on staying pain-free and active for life.

GET STRONGER (SAFELY) VERSUS JUST STRETCHING

While we lose both flexibility and strength as we age, contrary to what most people believe, preventing injuries and overcoming aches and pains is less about stretching or flexibility, and more about getting stronger. Many people (the prior me included) believe that if something is hurting, we must stop all activity and stretch out the painful area.

While stretching, massage, creams, heat, or ice can provide temporary relief, to truly avoid chronic pain, your focus has to be on strengthening the area and all of the surrounding muscles that support it. Not only does strengthening prevent aches and pains but also improves flexibility and allows us to move a joint through its full range of motion. This keeps us mobile as we age.

A classic example is the lower back, which is a very common ailment among over-40 professionals. In fact, I estimate that two thirds of my clients report lower back pain at some point. To beat lower back pain, it's important to strengthen the lower back, as well as all the muscles that support it including your core, hips, and hamstrings (all of which get overused and become tight from all of the sitting we do while we're working, driving, etc.).

But like I said, the exercises you choose have to be done safely, while challenging you enough to elevate your metabolism—you have to find the sweet spot.

To guide you in bulletproofing your body I've incorporated the six functional movement patterns prescribed for pain-free performance by my mentor, Dr. John Rusin in the

Strength Training Plan you will see in Chapter 19, "Shift #4: Train For Strength."

The strength training routine will challenge you but is safe to do because it works in alignment with how your body was designed to move. It will help you transform your body safely, even if you're over-40, aren't much of an athlete, have prior injuries, or are coming back from a long lay off.

If they helped my client Walter bounce back, they will work for you too.

QUICK ACTION

With all the sitting we do these days, lower back pain has become a common ailment. To avoid pain in this area we have to gradually strengthen the muscles that support the lower back. Namely, our core.

To strengthen your core, incorporate planks and glute bridges into your workouts or daily movement routine.

They're gentle and low in intensity. If you're not sure how to do them, check Google or YouTube.

Do these moves regularly to reduce back pain and prevent future aches.

PROGRAM MANAGER COLLABORATES TO OVERCOME MAJOR INJURY AND TRANSFORM IN MIND AND BODY

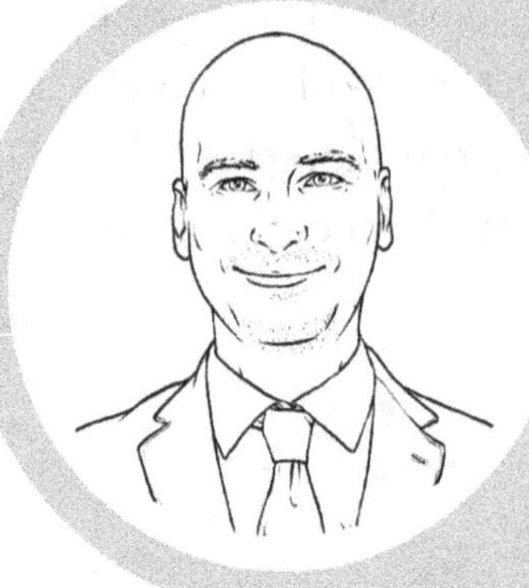

Never before had I had a mantra or an affirmation to keep me grounded. Something that you could always pull from to keep you focused on the goals.
–Walter

THE SITUATION

When Walter was in the military, he had a tribe of peers who would motivate and push one another to stay fit and healthy. When he transitioned to civilian life, he lost this support system. He turned to CrossFit for a period of time but was no longer able to perform its intense physical demands when a serious back injury required spinal fusion surgery. Limitations from this injury, combined with a period of high stress, hypothyroidism (Hashimoto's thyroiditis), and low testosterone, led to Walter gaining significant body fat, driving his weight up from 190 lb to 252 lb.

Walter's confidence and self-image were shattered, and he was terrified that if he didn't make a lasting change soon, he was going to become overly dependent on his family during old age and be a bad father. Like many high achievers, Walter demanded perfection from himself and was hard on himself when he didn't meet his own high standards.

THE SOLUTION

By crafting a plan that worked around the limitations that resulted from his back injury we helped Walter regain the confidence to move and exercise. Due to his work schedule and long commute, Walter also needed a plan that he could execute at home, without going to a gym. We set him up with home workouts he was able to do with minimal equipment. Monitoring his blood work and health markers, we made sure his previous thyroid and sex hormone imbalances were not impeding his progress.

We also worked with Walter to transform his mindset in order to be more trusting, in himself and the process, practice more self-love and acceptance, and give himself permission to do things that bring him more joy, like rebuilding his antique Corvette.

THE TRANSFORMATION

Walter was able to lose over 30 lb of fat in his first six months on the program and he built noticeable muscle. As a result of his transformation, he feels more accepting of himself, even when he's not being perfect. Walter has the mindset tools he relies on to create greater internal peace and stay grounded, even when his stress levels are high.

Regarding one of the mindset tools we gave him, he had this to say: "Never before had I had a mantra or an affirmation to keep me grounded. Something that you could always pull from to keep you focused on the goals. Those are way more powerful than people give them credit for."

Today, he fits and looks better in his clothes. This gave Walter the confidence to go out and secure a new job that he finds more fulfilling. It pays him more, too!

MIND

Emotional Eating
Limiting Beliefs
Wavering Motivation

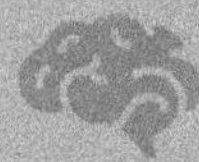

BODY

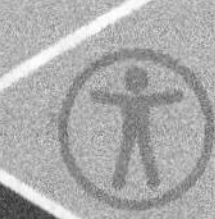

Slowing Metabolism
Changing Hormones
Injuries & Limitations

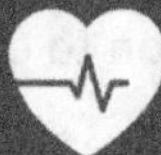

LIFE

High Stress

CHAPTER 10

CHALLENGE #7: High Stress

"Stress is the trash of modern life; we all generate it, but if you don't dispose of it properly, it will pile up and overtake your life."
—Danzae Pace

OK, we just wrapped up the body-related challenges of a slowing metabolism, changing hormones, and potential for injuries. Now, let's turn our attention to the third category of challenges: life.

An aspect of life is having to deal with stress; it's a common reality for all of us. Even more so if you're a professional over the age of forty.

Most professionals deal with daily stressors such as team meetings, budgeting, financial decisions, presentations, pitches, business travel, client calls, hiring and firing, legal situations, operational matters, or other important items. As a career professional, you are constantly undergoing stress—and that's just at work.

Next comes the stressors from family and personal life. Not to mention the internal stress caused by the lofty, and sometimes unforgiving, standards that make you a high achiever in the first place.

It's not just emotional stress that you deal with, either. Add in the potential stressors on the body itself, such as a crummy night's sleep, poor nutrition, alcohol, environmental toxins, jet lag—and you've got stressors coming at you from all directions.

Whether it's due to work or life, stress can make it harder to attain and maintain a body that is lean, strong, and energized.

UNDERSTANDING THE TYPES AND SOURCES OF STRESS

While entire books have been written about the topic of stress, for the purposes of mitigating this common obstacle to your body goals, let's briefly define what we mean by "stress" by categorizing it by its type and source.

The 2x2 Stress Matrix illustrates the types and sources of stress:

TYPES OF STRESS: ACUTE VS. CHRONIC

One way to categorize stress is by type, which is given by its duration.

Acute stress comes in short, sharp bursts, but usually goes away fairly quickly. Examples include the shock of an oncoming car, getting stunned by a loud noise, anger after an argument, panic after losing a wallet, or the despair of running to catch a flight whose boarding gate is about to close.

Chronic stress, on the other hand, can last longer and is ongoing. Examples include long-lasting emotional stress due

THE STRESS MATRIX

TYPE	SOURCE: Internal	SOURCE: External
Chronic	Fears Concerns Depression	Work Life
Acute	Shock Panic Illness	Sudden Threat Immediate Danger

to traumas, concerns about finances, workplace stress, challenging family dynamics, going through a divorce, or rooting for the Dallas Cowboys.

SOURCES OF STRESS: INTERNAL VS. EXTERNAL

Another way to categorize stress is by its source; stress can either come from the inside or the outside.

Internal stress is the self-imposed tension we experience that arises inside of us. This would include things like our judgements (about yourself and others), beliefs, opinions, fears, worries, anxieties, sadness, ruminations, regrets, apprehensions, or ambitions. If you recall, these are emotional stressors we covered in Chapter 4, "Challenge #1: Emotional Eating."

On the other hand, external stress happens outside of us and is usually out of our control. This would include things like traffic, the stock market, weather, or other people's behavior or their decisions.

Now, let's get clear on the physiological responses stress has on the body.

Fair warning: the effects of stress can be pretty nasty.

Effects of Stress On the Body

Besides leading to stress eating, the experience of stress on the body has many physiological effects that, if it endures and is not managed properly, can make it hard for us to maintain our body and health where we want them to be.

In basic terms, stress puts our nervous system into a sympathetic state, which is also known as our fight-or-flight response. This mechanism exists to help us survive. If not kept in check, chronic stress can lead to continuously elevated cortisol levels. This can result in numerous adaptations that can become deleterious to the body over time.

Persistent elevation of cortisol can lead to:

- further slowing of an already aging metabolism
- hormonal imbalances
- elevated blood sugar levels
- insulin resistance (IR) and the potential for diabetes
- disruption of gut health and digestion

In addition, elevated cortisol can trigger hunger cravings by elevating the hunger hormone ghrelin (causing overeating), or it can shut down our appetite by tanking our satiety hormone, leptin (also causing overeating). Furthermore, chronically elevated cortisol impairs cognitive function, hurting decision making and causing brain fog.

And I'm sorry to say . . . it gets even worse.

Consistently elevated cortisol does a double whammy on your skeletal muscle. First, it lowers testosterone levels, our key muscle building and fat-fighting hormone. Second, it eats into your existing muscle tissue. That's because cortisol breaks down both fat and muscle to produce the energy we need to deal with stress. A reduction in muscle tissue reduces your metabolism further, potentially leading to even more body fat, less energy, as well as decreased strength and mobility over time.

Is that nasty enough for you yet?

No?

OK, here's another one.

Chronically elevated cortisol, especially in the evenings, hampers the quality of your sleep by limiting melatonin production. Consequently, getting poor sleep triggers a vicious cycle that elevates cortisol and blood sugar levels even further the next day.

If chronically elevated cortisol due to mental or emotional stress persists too intensely or too long, it can cause a condition known as adrenal fatigue (as we covered in Chapter 8, "Challenge #5: Changing Hormones"). Its symptoms include constant tiredness, cravings for sugar or stimulants like caffeine, and disruption of sleep patterns.

Given all this, here's what's ironic . . .

Many high-achievers add fuel to the fire by trying to power their way to achieving their desired body by pushing themselves harder and harder. They will pursue restrictive diets or extreme workouts in the midst of everything else going on at work and at home.

What many fail to realize is that dieting and too much exercise are also sources of stress on the body that elevate cortisol and lead to fat gain and reduced muscle mass. If you've ever dieted very strictly or worked out really intensely but weren't seeing results, this can be a major reason why. (I feel some lightbulbs turning on right about now.)

Too much dieting and too much exercise are sources of stress on the body.

So, to put all this in simple terms: high stress, whether due to internal (emotional) or external (work or life-related) sources, can make it much harder for an over-40 professional to meet his or her body and health goals.

But stress isn't going away, so let's learn how to fight back against this sinister challenge, shall we?

THERE'S HOPE FOR DEALING WITH EXTERNAL STRESSORS

Needless to say, if we let outside influences cause us to react from a place of fear or ego, they can create negative outcomes for us, including feeling stressed and falling off of our habits.

HOW NICK'S INTENSE NEGOTIATIONS WOULD THROW OFF HIS ROUTINE

My client Nick is an investment banker who represents companies that are going through bankruptcy. When a corporation liquidates, it sells off its assets and distributes them to debt holders and then to shareholders according to the liquidation preference of those financial instruments. During such liquidations, most of the investors will only get back pennies on the dollar, while some won't even get a single penny.

Negotiations during liquidation proceedings can get quite tense, with angry investors and even government officials shooting blame, criticism, and accusations towards the failed company and its representatives. Having to be on the receiving end of these flaming arrows is Nick's job.

During these fiery negotiations, the opposing side tries to break down the defending side's arguments and win back as much money as possible from the failing corporation. Voices are raised, mind games are played, shouting can ensue, and sometimes insults even get hurled. Nick would take the brunt of these assaults.

These sessions would sometimes leave Nick not only exhausted, but emotionally worked up for days. As a result, his health habits would suffer. He'd cope with alcohol and other vices to recoup—this was in addition to the anti-anxiety meds he was already on.

Tense arguments and criticism can get us in our head and trigger our core limiting belief. For Nick, this would trigger his limiting belief of "I don't belong," which started when his family emigrated to the United States from the Czech Republic when Nick was ten years old. Being the new kid on the block, who didn't even speak English, in a U.S. school with kids that teased him made Nick feel like an outsider. His deep-seated fear of not belonging led him to take on the identity of a perfectionist. He sought to prove himself through good grades and impressive accomplishments like being accepted to an Ivy league school and getting recruited to work on Wall Street for a top investment bank. But they came at the price of anxiety and other health issues.

These negotiation sessions would trigger Nick's anxiety. His job was to look good in front of his clients and be able to defend them against the onslaught of angry investors. He'd often feel insecure in these settings, especially if the negotiations did not go well for him and his client.

For a high achieving perfectionist, failure is a very tough thing to accept because it threatens their survival strategy. Their accomplishments validate their worth, and when they can't "succeed" their way out of a situation, their old fears and limiting beliefs come rushing back.

For Nick, these meetings would put him in an anxious funk for days.

Now, you may or may not get paid big money to absorb the arrows of angry investors like Nick does for his clients. But we all have to deal with tense, or at least delicate, conversations at some point. These conversations can trigger us and throw us out of our groove. Naturally, when we experience inner stress it kills our motivation to do our health habits. We're much more likely to numb the pain with poor coping mechanisms like comfort foods, alcohol and other vices. Thus, we have to be able to protect ourselves from getting derailed by external stressors, such as tough conversations, so we can stay on track with our body transformation goals.

In Nick's case, I taught him a powerful mindset technique called "Recreating." It gives you the power to not be affected or triggered by what another person is saying to you. It will not only help you to not get stressed and thrown off of your health routine by what someone else is saying, but will also help you be much more effective in your interpersonal relationships, both at work and at home. Now, wouldn't that be a cool superpower to have?

Well, no worries. Because you're going to learn about this technique soon. (And that's "non-negotiable!")

Life happens and we have no control over it, but we have to learn how to respond effectively to outside influences so that they don't throw us off of our routine.

While it's easy to understand this concept at a logical level, just understanding it doesn't prevent us from getting triggered, distracted, or derailed by what happens. Just like with internal stress, what's required to manage external stress (caused by things that are out of our control) is to work at an emotional level. Specifically, having practices that keeps us in an empowered emotional state no matter what goes on around us. Otherwise, it can cause us to abandon our body transformation habits and lose momentum.

These practices can create a "stress shield" to keep us grounded and prevent us from abandoning our habits when external stressors hit.

A simple daily practice that creates a positive emotional state can create a "stress shield" against external stressors and prevent us from getting triggered.

Now, this doesn't mean by doing certain practices we'll never ever get triggered or upset or get knocked off of our routine. After all, most of us are not monks or stoic philosophers. We'll inevitably get triggered at some point. The goal is to reduce the frequency and impact of outside events on our internal stress levels. We can accomplish this with the right empowerment practices. You will learn some great ones when we get to Chapter 23, "Shift #7: Mitigate External Stressors." For now, here's a quick one you can try.

QUICK ACTION

An effective and enjoyable way to stay more grounded and resilient against external stress is to replenish your "emotional bank account" regularly. One way to do that is to do what my cousin Emanuela and I call "feeding your soul." Do something simple that brings you joy, and do it regularly.

Pick one or two things you will do each week to fill up your emotional bank account:

- listening to your favorite music
- calling your best friend
- playing with a child or a pet
- filling up a scrapbook
- watching your favorite movie
- taking a walk in a place you love
- flying a kite
- riding a bike
- dancing
- painting
- drawing
- writing
- playing a video game
- playing a instrument
- playing a sport

Anything active or creative is great, but really, it can be anything that truly brings you joy. (Yes, anything. No judgments!)

DOCTOR FINDS THE CURE FOR HIGH STRESS AND WEIGHT GAIN

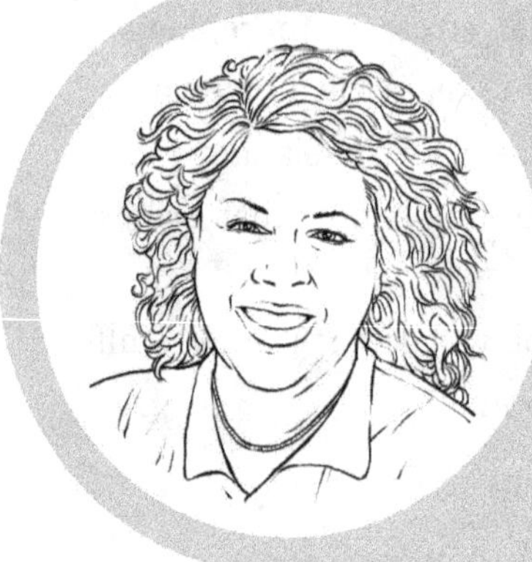

I don't know how I got this bad, but I have to get back to my old self!
–Diana

THE SITUATION

Even though she was active for most of her life, Diana had gained weight during a period of high stress. Her weight had gone from 140 lb up to 195 lb, and she was distraught. At this weight, Diana didn't feel good in her skin, and was concerned about her health. Worse for her was the fact she had lost the mobility needed to play sports with her kids. She sorely missed going rollerblading and skiing with them.

"I don't know how I got this bad, but I have to get back to my old self!" she vented.

Diana had tried to get the weight down through walking and fitness classes but progress was slow; she was struggling and felt stuck. Between running her private practice, community events, and parenting, her schedule was constantly full, leaving her little time to exercise and eat structured, healthy meals. She wanted to get her health habits done in a way that was enjoyable but did not disrupt her ability to fulfill her numerous work and life responsibilities.

Diana's goal? "To age like Angela Bassett," by staying sexy and strong into her 60s and beyond.

THE SOLUTION

First, we coached her on how to stay motivated and keep momentum up, even when overwhelm or apathy would kick in.

Then, we crafted Diana a very flexible routine that she could adapt to her limited and constantly changing schedule. We struck a balance between doing workouts that would effectively boost her metabolism and burn fat, and doing activities she enjoyed, like jumping rope and attending her weekend kickboxing class. We also gave Diana numerous nutrition strategies she could incorporate on the fly and adapt to her changing schedule of patients.

THE TRANSFORMATION

In the course of six months, Diana lost 50 lb, going from 195 lb to 145 lb.

She felt very relieved at having gotten unstuck and back to her normal self. This gave her tremendous self-confidence and a feeling of accomplishment. For Diana, the biggest win was the fact she was able to go skiing again with her kids. Plus, she was also happy to set an example for her best friend and others in her community.

She was so ecstatic and "over the moon" about her transformation you can say that her exit interview with us was filled with pretty colorful, NSFW, language. (In a good effing way!)

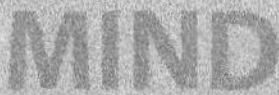

MIND

Emotional Eating
Limiting Beliefs
Wavering Motivation

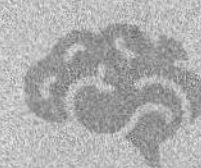

BODY

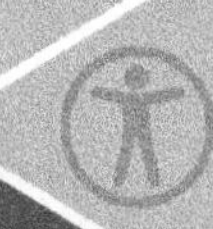

Slowing Metabolism
Changing Hormones
Injuries & Limitations

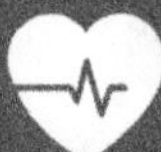

LIFE

High Stress
Limited Time

CHAPTER 11

CHALLENGE #8: Limited Time

"My favorite things in life don't cost any money. It's really clear that the most precious resource we all have is time."
—Steve Jobs

Pretty sure I'm not going out on a limb by saying that you rarely have enough time to do everything you'd like to do.

Whether it's a packed work calendar, family obligations, social commitments, or business travel (more on that later), time is usually the one resource we rarely have enough of. I see it all the time with my clients:

- Stacy, an executive director of sales at a SaaS provider, is booked on back-to-back Zoom calls all day, every day. She rarely finds the time to sit down and eat a proper meal.
- Christopher, a corporate litigation attorney in New York City, has to put in 100-hour weeks when preparing for a trial.

- Tammy, a senior finance executive, is buried under the workload left behind by a colleague who quit unexpectedly, leaving Tammy without enough time or energy to get her workouts in each night.

You, undoubtedly, have a packed schedule as well.

When our schedules get filled with work, family, and other obligations, the first thing we tend to cut out is our health habits. I was guilty of this, too, whenever I got busy. That's one big reason why it took me so long to break through my struggles and achieve my goals in a lasting way.

A typical week for me when I was working as a strategy consultant would look like this: put in 60–80 hours at work on a consulting engagement, usually out of town. I'd fly out Monday mornings (early) and fly back home on Thursday night (late). Saturday was dedicated to errands and date night with the wife. Sunday was brunch with friends in the Upper West Side near Central Park, or a visit with family. Before I knew it, Sunday night would sneak up on me and I'd have to pack for another work trip in the morning.

As a high achiever, I'm sure your weeks are just as busy, if not more.

OUR BELIEFS ABOUT TIME

What stops a lot of people is they buy into limiting beliefs that they "have no time" or that they're just "too busy" to worry about trying to lose weight or optimize their body. So they don't even bother trying.

Remember, the mind draws its conclusions and beliefs from evidence. When we don't do something for an extended period, evidence starts to mount that it can't be done. Fortunately, the opposite is also true. Once we start proving to our mind that it ***can*** be done, it starts to believe it and act accordingly. So, the secret then, is to find efficient ways to get your routine done, no matter how busy you might be.

Take, for example, my client, Larry, a 50-year old project manager for IBM who is married with two kids and has a passion for singing. He has a full work and life schedule to say the least. In his first twelve weeks on our program, which were summer months, he was regularly taking his kids up to camp on the weekends and he'd perform with his band while he was up there. On top of this, he traveled for work several times, went on a cruise with his wife, and then spent a full week celebrating his fiftieth birthday (and didn't "hold back" very much). In spite of all this, he was still able to fit in the efficient habits we taught him to lose over a pound per week—fifteen pounds total—during these first twelve (very busy) weeks on our program. And that was despite dealing with bad knees, a bad back, and elevated A1C.

Now, I don't want to be lame and use the old cliche "If he can do it, anyone can." The point of the story, though, is even with a full work and life schedule, it's still possible to find a minimal amount of time to balance out your health habits and get them done. The catch is to make the most of that time you are spending.

EFFICIENCY ENSURES CONSISTENCY

There are a number of factors that make it hard to get our habits done efficiently and consistently. Like we've been saying, it could be due to mental challenges like our emotions, limiting beliefs, and wavering motivation. It can also be due to the demands on our time that life, and other people, throw our way.

Because these demands result in us having limited time, many over-40 professionals end up either skipping out on their habits, or doing them but spending a long time for paltry results. Alternating between these two extremes can be discouraging. It can make us feel like we're wasting our valuable time or that it's simply not possible to have the body we want given our busy schedule. These conclusions can sink our motivation, cause inconsistency, or make us want to quit altogether.

Pointing to reasons why you don't have enough time will give your subconscious mind all the evidence it needs to make it true and keep you consistently short on time.

When our time is limited, we need to be efficient and take control of the situation. But instead of being proactive, people fall prey to common mistakes.

First, they don't properly schedule their habits in their calendar and leave things to chance. They also don't communicate the times set aside for their habits to those around them. This can often lead to the dreaded "double booking" when people schedule us to do something when we were supposed to be doing something for our health, like exercising.

Second, they don't create the space and the "me time" needed to actually do their habits by establishing boundaries for these times. (People pleasers, I'm looking at you.) By not saying "no" and protecting the time we need for our self-care when we're supposed to (like when we agree to work late even though we were supposed to get a workout in that night), we increase the chance of getting overwhelmed and falling off of our body transformation habits.

Third, they spend too much time doing low-value activities (like a lot of walking or cardio classes), which only deliver a small benefit when it comes to trying to transform your body quickly.

In an age when we're busier—and unhealthier—than ever, it's essential to get good at balancing our health habits with everything pulling at us. Because going non-stop without maintaining at least a minimum level of consistency in our health habits will inevitably lead to a decline in our body, health, performance, and, inevitably, our quality of life.

Obviously, we may sometimes have a crisis that requires our attention for a few days or even a few weeks. Skipping some workouts to deal with urgent matters like handling an important work deadline, moving our home, caring for a sick child, or grieving the loss of a loved one is not only understandable, it's prudent. But if running non-stop and ignoring our health habits becomes the norm for too long, it becomes unsustainable and we will eventually pay the price with our health and happiness.

The more efficient we can make our habits, the more it ensures we do them consistently. In fact, taking a more efficient approach to our body transformation not only saves us time, but also reduces resistance. That's because the more time and effort we have to spend on something, the more our mind's comfort zone will chime in and put up a fight. According to Joey Thurman, author of *The Minimum Method*,[31] instead of taking the approach of "no pain, no gain," which can feel daunting, he states that "there can actually be benefits to giving minimal effort . . . minimum effort can actually be more effective than maximum effort. Our goal is efficiency, the least effort for the most gain." I fully agree, and will add that the more efficient we can be from a time, focus, and exertion standpoint, the greater the chance our mind will not resist or derail us from staying consistent with our habits over time.

THERE'S HOPE FOR DEALING WITH LIMITED TIME

If you've struggled with not having enough time, know that there is good news. *The Nine Shifts* was designed to be efficient so you can get your habits in quickly. It's also flexible so you can maintain your progress even when life gets crazy.

You only need to invest 3–5 hours per week to keep your body and health optimal. That's just about four percent of your waking hours.

It may be hard for some folks to believe, but once you get into a groove, that's really all the time it takes to keep the (right) habits that will keep your metabolism high, your body lean, and your energy primed. The Keep Efficient Habits Plan in Chapter 24 will show you exactly how to do this. For now, here's a simple way to become more efficient.

QUICK ACTION

Here's an important tool called "imperfect actions." Not only do imperfect actions help you get out of limiting beliefs and demotivation due to their simple, doable nature, but also save you time because they're highly efficient. As an example, my client Faith travels a ton, and one thing I taught her to do was walk around the terminal while she's waiting for her flight to board, instead of sitting at the gate like everyone else.

Ask yourself, "What imperfect actions can I take today that would not require me spending any more time?" Some suggestion include:

- Can I stand instead of sitting during a Zoom call?
- Can I have a meeting with someone while walking at the same time?
- Can I take a call and combine it with a post-meal walk (to elevate my metabolism and improve digestion) before getting back to work or other responsibilities?

You can get as creative as you like. Some people will do things like get a standing desk, walk on a treadmill while working or studying, or purposely take the stairs instead of the elevator. All of these are examples of getting in motion without requiring any dedicated time out of your schedule.

NYC ATTORNEY NO LONGER "SENTENCED" TO GAINING BODY FAT DURING CRUNCH TIME

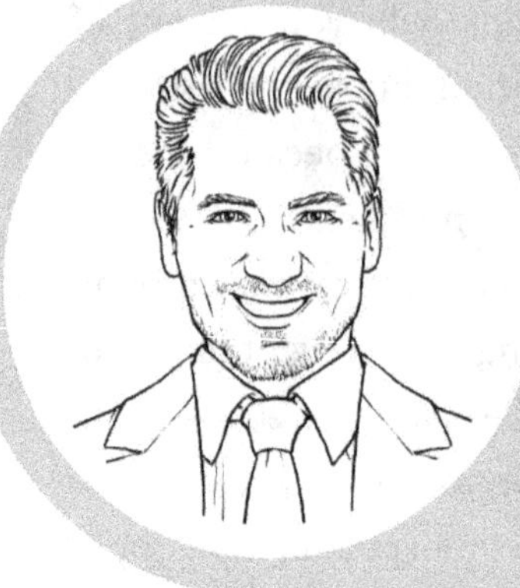

Thanks to you, I've eaten clean and had the tools around me so I was able to continue to be healthy when life became very unhealthy.

–Christopher

THE SITUATION

Christopher is a high-powered attorney who helps multinational corporations through crises like bankruptcy and restructuring. His work often requires him to represent his clients in litigation, and when he's preparing for court proceedings, he can work over a hundred hours in a week. The double-whammy of high stress and limited sleep used to cause Christopher to gain body fat when his workload soared like this. As a result, his body fat percentage kept creeping up until it hit 27%. He wasn't technically overweight or obese, but Christopher didn't like how he looked and wanted to carry himself with more confidence. Christopher had tried all the tricks he'd learned in his younger days as an athlete—tracking calories, steps, sleep, and other metrics—but it wasn't giving him the change he wanted.

THE SOLUTION

Christoper was highly driven, so mindset and motivation were not an issue. With him, we moved right into optimization of his body and life. Because he is a data junkie, we took a metrics-based approach to show him, scientifically, the numbers around what, when, and how much to eat, as well as how to track and measure sleep and body composition metrics. We created a streamlined weekly exercise routine for when work was stable, and hyper-efficient strategies to maintain his progress when he had to put in 100-hour weeks. We also gave Christopher custom strategies and convenient nutrition sources to get his macronutrients in between meetings when work got intense. Finally, we recommended that he put a greater emphasis on strength training to efficiently increase his metabolism and burn more fat around the clock, even while billing clients!

THE TRANSFORMATION

These strategies had a profound effect on Christopher! In just a few short months he was able to reduce his body fat from 27% to nearly 20% while adding noticeable muscle mass. Best of all, he was able to keep his weight, even during his most hectic weeks.

But that's not all. Thanks to consistently maintaining his strength at a high level and his nutrition optimized, he recently started beating his squash instructor in matches, something he could never do before. I guess you can say Christopher has become the king of the "court," in more ways than one!

What I'm personally most proud of is the difference we were able to make for him in navigating what he described to be one of the most intense stretches of his career. He had this to say:

"I've not slept very much in the past 72 hours. Insane/brutal time at work. Worked from 6pm Friday to 3am Sunday nonstop, then got up at 5am and just finished at 11pm. Hopefully this week will get easier. Stress at insane levels, but taking the supplements I have for this situation. Just letting you guys know that what you do makes a big difference. Thank you."

Emotional Eating
Limiting Beliefs
Wavering Motivation

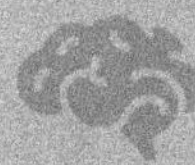

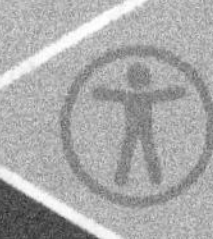

BODY
Slowing Metabolism
Changing Hormones
Injuries & Limitations

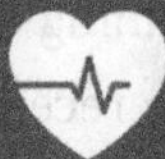

LIFE
High Stress
Limited Time
Travel & Social

CHAPTER 12

CHALLENGE #9: Travel & Social

"One can travel this world and see nothing. To achieve understanding it is necessary not to see many things, but to look hard at what you do see."
—Georgio Morandi

Traveling or attending social events represent situations where things like food and time are out of our control. As such, they can make it harder to stay on track with our body transformation habits. Some of us travel more than others, but when it comes to social events like weddings, birthday parties, or family gatherings, those events affect almost all of us. (Except for those of us living in a bubble, like I sometimes wish I could!)

So, let's first dive into the challenges that social events can pose to our waistline and health. Then, we'll tackle the challenges my fellow road warriors face.

SOCIAL EVENTS

Human beings are social creatures. The bonds we build with others are essential to happiness and life satisfaction. Studies have shown that maintaining social connections are important for stress reduction, mental health, longevity, and overall happiness. Indeed, being around our tribe is a subconscious survival tactic handed down from our ancestors. That's because our tribe would provide us with protection from other tribes or pillagers.

That being said, social events are notorious for having an abundance of rich foods and drinks, and the peer pressure to indulge in them. Whether it's with friends, family, or a work dinner, the expectation to eat and not be rude is very real.

If not managed carefully, social events can start affecting our waistline, especially if they occur too many days in a row. Some people are great all week and then totally go off the rails on the weekends, attending happy hours, date nights, social gatherings, nightclubs, concerts, sports events, brunches, etc.

If that doesn't affect you, then maybe you're faced with other types of events like weddings, birthdays, BBQs, potlucks, or the holidays. A study by *The New England Journal of Medicine* revealed that close to 70% of Americans expect to gain weight (between 5–15 lb during the holidays), while 62% said they would skip a holiday party to avoid food temptations.[32]

When it comes to social events, we want to find a way to have our (birthday) cake and eat it too. This goal is to learn how to attend them, and enjoy them, without them adversely affecting our body and health.

Our mind's wiring compels us to follow social norms, even if they're not the healthiest for us.

Like with all of the challenges we may face, let's start with how the mind will play a role. One of the ways the mind tries to ensure your survival is by winning the acceptance and protection of your tribe. So it will do its best to fit in by not breaking social norms or allow you to look bad in front of the group. This means not being the "weird one" who won't eat or drink like the others. For instance, saying you're on a "diet" and not eating usually gets pushback from friends. Refusing food or drink when visiting someone's home can be seen as rude.

I, myself, feel the peer pressure. I drink little to no alcohol, and that makes things hard in a very alcohol-focused culture. Try going to a bar and ordering something non-alcoholic. The options are very limited. I also stay away from sugary drinks like sodas and juices due to their tendency to spike blood sugar levels and insulin. Now, my options are even more limited.

Worse, it sets up a strange dynamic. You want to be with your friends and be social, but you don't want to drink. They're getting merry while you're still sober. Some of them try to con or shame you into drinking. Others are actually happy that you're not drinking because you can be their designated driver.

If I meet a date for a drink, it becomes nearly impossible to not have alcohol. Getting her a drink while you drink water is not exactly the best way to make a good first impression.

All this to say, social norms around eating and drinking create both subconscious pressure and peer pressure to consume things that are not the healthiest for us or in line with our goals. I'm sure we've all gone to weddings, or holiday feasts, or have had too many nights in a row of being social where we emerged feeling less than great about our choices because we were wrapped up in the moment or went with the flow of the group.

This applies to both personal situations and to work settings. I remember that at one point, two of my high-achieving clients—one a high-powered attorney and the other an investment banker—attended the same work conference. They said everyone there, besides them, were not only unhealthy looking but also were carelessly indulging in rich foods and alcohol over the course of the three-day event. (I have to say I was proud of my "boys" for having the courage to stand out and do their best to stay balanced and disciplined in such a challenging social environment; it brought a tear to my eye!)

BEING SMARTER WITH ALCOHOL GUIDE

The next time you're out at a social event, keep this alcohol strategy in mind.

Your best option will always be clear liquor (vodka, gin, tequila blanco) mixed in club soda, with a simple garnish like lemon, lime, orange, or cucumber slices. Not the most exciting, I know, but easiest on the waistline.

Don't shoot the messenger, but I recommend limiting or skipping the following drinks:

- **Beer:** Has gluten, which can be inflammatory. It also elevates estrogen, which can cause us to store more body fat. (And you thought beer was what "real men" drink!) If you do drink beer, know that light beer will save you about 40 calories per 12 oz serving versus regular beer.
- **Wine:** While the antioxidants in wine can be helpful in moderation, wine also contains sulfites, which can trigger allergies in some people. Red wines are higher in histamines, which can trigger reactions like itching, headaches, or indigestion in select populations. Non-red wines can be a better option as far as it being easier on the body, just note that both red and white wine have about the same number of calories per glass, approximately 120.
- **Mixed or Frozen Drinks:** This includes drinks like a margarita, mojito, Moscow Mule, Cosmo, Rum & Coke, etc. Mixed or frozen drinks (and tonics) are usually high in sugar and calories. In fact, a Piña Colada has close to 600 calories (Wow!). Sugary drinks create a rush of fast-burning carbs that our body can not use quickly enough. The result is a spike in insulin and the likely storage of that energy as body fat.

FREQUENT TRAVEL AND BEING AWAY FROM HOME

For many professionals, frequent travel is a way of life. My client Ron is a Two-Million Miler on Delta and a Million-Miler on United. Needless to say, he travels ***a lot*** for work, flying from the West Coast to the East Coast, and back, on a regular basis. Another client of mine, Faith, would fly from the Midwest, where she worked, to Orlando every weekend to tend to her aging mom. Deborah, a real estate agency owner who is constantly meeting clients, doing showings, and evaluating properties, is away from home on a daily basis.

Whether you spend a lot of time in airports or around town, being away from home can make it more challenging to maintain the health habits that keep you optimal. To say that the pre-packaged food items or fast food meals that we find at airports, truck stops, convenience stores, pharmacies, and gas stations are not great for us might be one of the greatest understatements of the year.

Do you drive around town much? Depending on which part of the U.S. you live, driving around daily can lure you into a web of convenient, grab-and-go, pre-packaged, and processed food options that will subtly push you further down the slippery slope of poor health. Ever go to trade shows? Don't even get me started about the food options at expo halls. Ever attended sporting events or shows with clients of friends? Fuggedaboudit!

Traveling also creates challenges in other ways. Business trips usually mean long, stressful days that include compulsory on-site lunches, lavish dinners with clients, and free-flowing wine and drink. The social norms and peer pressure to consume in these settings comes with the territory.

"Frequent business travelers have a 260% greater likelihood of rating their health as fair to poor, compared with light travelers."[33]

Besides the aforementioned nutrition curveballs, traveling makes exercising harder too. Hotels are very hit-or-miss when it comes to their fitness centers. If you can even find the time to squeeze in a workout during your packed days on the road, that is.

Traveling for personal trips isn't any less challenging.

The high stress of work and life can tempt us to let loose during vacations, which can make practicing discipline on personal trips very difficult. Second, most people like to experience new foods and drinks when vacationing (and rightfully so). I mean, you don't go all the way to Paris and not have some fine French wine and cheese, or go to Italy and not taste the yummy gelato, or go to Texas and not have some sizzling brisket. I'll be the first to admit that experiencing rich foods and drinks while on vacation is a treat that we'd be crazy not to enjoy. However, it can make things more challenging if you're looking to consistently keep your body and health in an optimal state.

I had one client, a pediatrician, who went on a two-week vacation to Cabo and really let loose. Suffice it to say he thoroughly enjoyed himself. To my horror, he came back almost fifteen pounds heavier, wiping out nearly all of the progress he had made during his first two months in my program. (Yikes!)

What's more, staying with friends or family while traveling adds the element of social norms. Good luck saying "no" to their savory home-cooked meals, toasts to your health, or grandma's heirloom apple pie. (Nor would I advise you to piss off grandma.)

In a nutshell, like with being at social events, being away from your kitchen and your exercise equipment due to travel can make it harder to stay consistent with your body transformation habits. Your goal is to find a way to easily withstand a few days of being less than perfect with your habits during work trips or vacations.

THERE'S HOPE FOR OVERCOMING TRAVEL & SOCIAL CHALLENGES

In summary, trips and vacations make it harder to stick to our routine and too many social events, like around the holidays, cause most people to gain weight. Travel and social events throw us curve balls that make it hard for us to stick to our usual habits. Poor quality food at airports and lack of workout equipment when traveling make it harder to stick to our routine. Social norms to eat rich foods and drink alcohol make it harder on our waistline.

These situations are inevitable. They're also delicate in terms of fitting in with social expectations. We don't want to be set back by them. Thus, it's essential to be prepared and have a plan to traverse them successfully so they don't cause us to break momentum with our habits.

QUICK ACTION

I teach my clients several techniques for minimizing the impact of alcohol on their waistline when they go to social events. One of these techniques I teach is what I called the Half-Tank Strategy.

In essence, you eat a little something before drinking alcohol. Having a bit of food in your stomach and "filling up halfway" will blunt the effects of any alcohol you might consume early on in the event. This helps from both an insulin-spiking aspect, as well as improving sobriety. Because, as we know, once that goes, our self-restraint around eating and drinking usually goes with it. (I can certainly attest to that from my younger days!)

Before you go out to a happy hour or dinner event, try out the Half-Tank strategy to prevent drinking on an empty stomach, or over-indulging on rich foods at the event.

Above all, enjoy and be safe!

SALES LEADER LEARNS HOW TO MEET HER HABIT QUOTA AND STAY OPTIMAL DURING WORK TRIPS

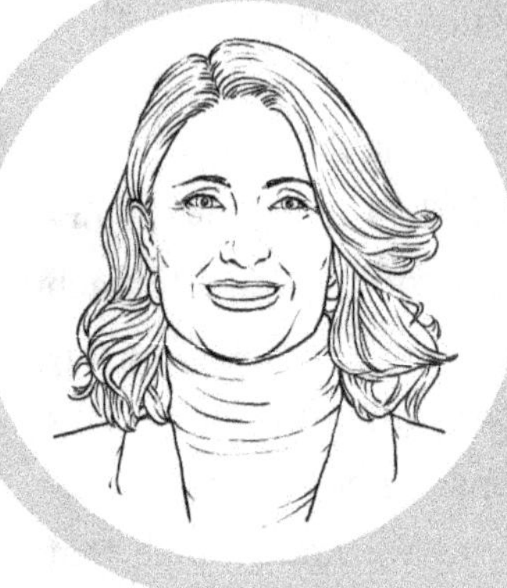

***The Nine Shifts* gave me a good plan that felt doable. It's not an overnight bullet. It's solid guidance on how you lose weight and increase your metabolism. –Stacy**

THE SITUATION

My client Stacy is Executive Director of Strategic Accounts at a SaaS provider. A lot of her sales calls happen face-to-face and this requires her to be on the road often. When she's on business trips, she's hustling from one client meeting to the next. As you can probably imagine (or relate), this makes her eating situation fairly unpredictable.

Sometimes she doesn't have much time to eat in between meetings. Other times, she's obligated to eat at the client appointment because the client may provide lunch, or Stacy may cater the lunch. These catered lunches are not always the healthiest. Moreover, she often hosts or attends client dinners, creating another situation where rich food or drinks will be present.

THE SOLUTION

To help create some predictability, we have Stacy start her day with a fairly hearty, high-protein meal at breakfast to kickstart her metabolism and start fulfilling her daily macronutrient goals before the madness begins.

Additionally, she keeps her Stay Optimal Travel Kit in hand (you'll learn about this essential travel tool in Chapter 25). It includes our plan-approved energy bars, protein powder, nuts, and other snacks and supplements to help backfill some of the macronutrients on days she won't get proper meals in due to her back-to-back meetings.

On days she knows for sure she will be meeting a client for dinner, she will sometimes do some fasting for part of the day to leave enough calorie budget to splurge a bit at the restaurant that night. We also give her a lower macro target to hit while traveling since it's harder to eat a lot while traveling.

For exercise, we taught her to stay fluid and get in whatever minimum level of activity her schedule allows. When she has the time and a good gym in her hotel, she starts her day by getting in a good workout. Other times, she has to do a quick resistance band workout using our workout app before she showers and heads out for the day. During those times that she gets little to no exercise during a trip, we encourage her to intentionally do some walking in the airport terminal while waiting for her plane to board.

When she returns from her trips and has some stability for a few days or weeks, we ramp up her workouts, macros, and calories to uplevel her metabolism.

THE TRANSFORMATION

Stacy was able to be successful using these strategies to transform her body—she lost 30 lb, got lean, tone, and got a flat and shapely stomach. This was despite the challenges of constant travel. She now has the tools to ensure her frequent business trips never set her back again. Here's what she had to say:

"I was allowing my job (and all the traveling I was doing) to run my life. I didn't feel healthy. I had tried diets and cardio but it felt insurmountable. *The Nine Shifts* has been life-changing!"

PART III

The Solution

CHAPTER 13

Introducing the Nine Shifts

"Simplicity is complexity resolved."
—Constantin Brancusi

So, what did you think of those nine challenges you just read about? Did you identify with some of them? Have they stopped you in trying to transform your body in a lasting way?

Perhaps by reading about the clients I featured you were able to relate to some of their previous frustrations. My wish is that you connected with their story, got inspired by how they overcame their obstacles, and now, you're inspired to overcome your own struggles too.

And overcome them, you will!

Just know that it's not easy.

WHY MOST PEOPLE STRUGGLE TO CONQUER THE NINE CHALLENGES

Those nine challenges are not only common for an over-40 professional, they're hard to surmount; they stop most people in their tracks. When these challenges stop us from getting our body to where we want it, we're dealt with a cruel blow—years spent being less than our best. Settling for a lower quality of life. Wishing and wondering how we can turn things around.

Compounding these challenges are two important factors.

First, most people aren't proficient in the domain of permanent body transformation and they make mistakes. They get thrown off mentally (by things like stress or low motivation), they work against their body (by doing things like dieting or the wrong exercises), or they don't account for life's obstacles (and get set back by work trips, holidays, and social events).

Second, the products and solutions out there simply aren't cutting it. There are more supplements, diet books, workout videos, cardio machines, activity trackers, fitness influencers, online coaches, hormone clinics, and personal trainers than ever before. Meanwhile, as a society, we're fatter, unhealthier, more depressed, and more diabetic than at any time in recorded history.

How can this be?

WHY MOST SOLUTIONS DON'T WORK VERY WELL

As mentioned in Chapter 1, "Why We Struggle," there are a slew of issues with this industry, especially in the realm of "weight loss," but here are the most problematic ones I see:

1. MOST SOLUTIONS ARE TEMPORARY (NO FOCUS ON LONG TERM BEHAVIOR CHANGE)

Do that 7-day Cleanse, 21-day Fat Loss Challenge, or 6-week Bootcamp and you know it's going to end. The expiration date is in the product name. Even things like monthly weight loss shake kits, pre-packaged "calorie controlled" meals in a monthly box, or some sessions with a personal trainer we will stop using at some point. What happens when they end? Well, we're back to square one, with pretty much the same old thoughts, stressors, and habits we had previously. When these come back, so does our old body.

2. TOO MUCH RANDOM AND GENERIC INFORMATION (WHICH LEADS TO CONFUSION)

While it's great that today we have access to tons of information about topics like nutrition, sleep, and losing weight, it also creates problems. First, it makes it hard to piece all that information together in a relevant way, and that's if it's all credible (which is a big "if"). Second, taking random advice because you "heard" something might work is not exactly a scientific approach to an area that requires applying some science. Sure, your coworker might have lost weight by doing intermittent fasting, but trying a random strategy in a vacuum without considering your diet history, current metabolic state, or circumstances can do more harm than good. Third, it can set the wrong goals and expectations. Why be lured into trying to, say, get shredded or have a six-pack like some influencer you just saw when, in reality, their genes are superior, they have lots of time to train, and are taking testosterone injections?

3. MOST SOLUTIONS ARE TOO NARROW (DON'T ACCOUNT FOR ALL THE ASPECTS)

When you were reading about the nine challenges, I'm willing to bet that you probably identified with more than one challenge. This is common. As you may recall, Tammy came to us post-menopausal with a slow metabolism, depression, and a lack of motivation. Tracy was dealing with high insulin levels and emotional eating. Chris was slammed with 100-hour weeks and constant travel. While it's good to seek help from professionals like hormone specialists, nutritionists, or personal trainers, and while there's nothing wrong with investing in cardio machines or a meal plan service, understand that they only deal with one narrow aspect of your transformation. They don't address all of it, nor do they account for the obstacles work or life may throw at you like high stress, a packed schedule, or traveling often.

Overall, while some of these solutions may get you some progress in the short term, few, if any, set you up in a way to see lasting results and ensure you maintain your results for life. Most of them leave us disappointed and searching for more answers. (Trust me, I know. I've tried many of them.)

LET'S TAKE A MORE COMPLETE AND LONG-LASTING APPROACH

I believe that people deserve something better. Call me crazy or overly-ambitious if you'd like (you wouldn't be the first!) but my goal is to plug the holes in this industry and give people something that is superior, by far. Something that helps them overcome all of the challenges standing in the way of achieving the body, health, and life they seek. Something that is truly:

- mindset-focused, to create long-term behavior change from the inside-out
- science-focused, to be relevant for a professional over-40
- holistic-focused, to be comprehensive and sustainable for life

I say:

Let's strive for more than quick fixes, gimmicks, and instant gratification.

Let's do better than temporary, narrow solutions.

Let's end confusion, guessing, and suffering.

Let's go beyond information . . .

. . . to achieve a true, lasting, and life-changing transformation!

ENTER THE NINE SHIFTS

I genuinely believe that my body transformation framework called *The Nine Shifts* helps solve many of the shortcomings

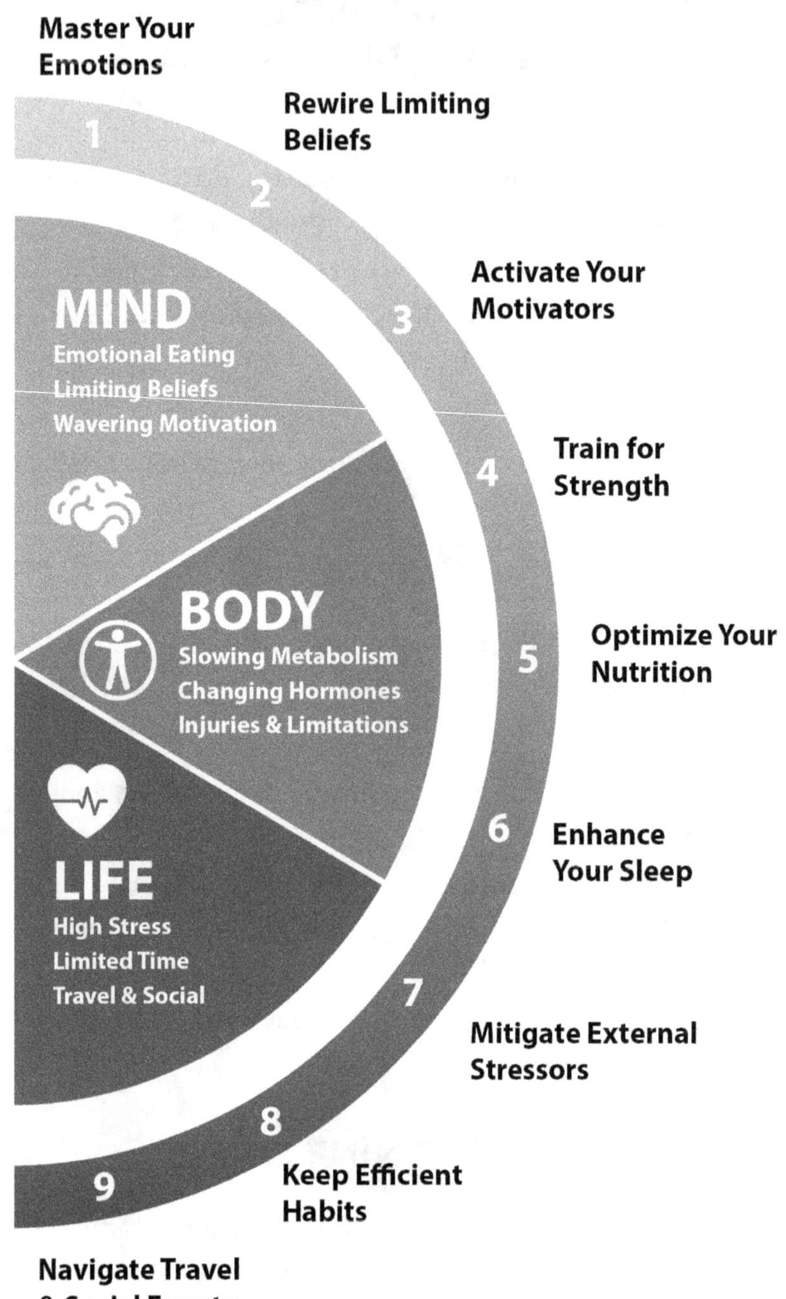
Master Your Emotions
Rewire Limiting Beliefs
Activate Your Motivators
Train for Strength
Optimize Your Nutrition
Enhance Your Sleep
Mitigate External Stressors
Keep Efficient Habits
Navigate Travel & Social Events
1
2
3
4
5
6
7
8
9
MIND
Emotional Eating
Limiting Beliefs
Wavering Motivation
BODY
Slowing Metabolism
Changing Hormones
Injuries & Limitations
LIFE
High Stress
Limited Time
Travel & Social

of most approaches and solutions. It's truly better than what people have been waiting for.

I'm about to reveal it to you, but before I do, I want to acknowledge you. You deserve a pat on the back for not giving up on achieving your potential and living your best life. Challenges may have stopped you, products and services may have failed you, but here you are, open to learning and trying something new. That takes courage and commitment. Most people would've quit by now. So for that, let me give you kudos.

Alright, now. Let's talk about conquering those pesky challenges and finally achieving long-term change!

The Nine Shifts is a framework that delivers a lasting transformation in your mind, body and life. It's designed with the over-40 professional in mind (but, really, can be used by anyone to achieve body success, whether they're twenty-five or seventy-five). These nine specific, carefully chosen shifts have come out of my desire to help people overcome the challenges and obstacles standing in the way of them achieving the body, health, and performance they desire. *The Nine Shifts* are for people—normal, everyday, very busy people—who want a no-BS, complete solution that takes them directly to their goals and keeps them there for good.

As you may remember from my transformation story earlier in the book, I designed the shifts after years of studying the science, working with top coaches, doing a ton of research, and rubbing elbows with professional bodybuilders. I took all of that information, boiled it down to the essentials and then tried it out with myself and then with some of my more adventurous clients. I stripped away the extra and figured out the real reasons why people weren't successful at achieving their health goals. Once I found those nine things, I rolled it out to the rest of my clients and saw it work for them, time and time again.

The Nine Shifts framework is designed to be practical, sustainable, and highly efficient. This way, it can become a part of your ongoing lifestyle.

As you can see from the diagram above, each challenge category—Mind, Body, Life—has a corresponding shift category that solves it – Mindset, Metabolism, Momentum. Here's a bit more about how it works.

MIND

To overcome the mind-related challenges of emotional eating, limiting beliefs, and wavering motivation you will make three shifts under the category of Mindset:

- Shift #1: Master Internal Stress
- Shift #2: Rewire Limiting Beliefs
- Shift #3: Activate Your Motivators

These shifts will empower you to gain deeper self-awareness so you can achieve greater calm, clarity and overall happiness. Along the way, you will learn to process negative emotions in a healthy way, become aware of how old beliefs are keeping you stuck, and gain the skills to maintain your motivation so you can be consistent with your body transformation habits.

The mindset shifts come first, because, as mentioned, *The Nine Shifts* is designed as a "mind-first" method to give you the foundation for achieving a true inside-out, total transformation. We'll be talking about that more deeply in the upcoming chapters.

BODY

To overcome the body-related challenges of a slowing metabolism, changing hormones, and injuries, you will make three shifts under the category of Metabolism:

- Shift #4: Train for Strength
- Shift #5: Optimize Your Nutrition
- Shift #6: Enhance Your Sleep

Obviously, no book about health and fitness would be complete without addressing the body. As you know now, being able to keep our metabolism high, especially as we age, gives your body the best chance of staying lean, healthy, and energized over the long run.

LIFE

To overcome the life-related challenges of high stress, limited time, and travel or social events, you will make three shifts under the category of Momentum:

- Shift #7: Mitigate External Stressors
- Shift #8: Keep Efficient Habits
- Shift #9: Navigate Travel & Social Events

This third shift category is also vital because it helps impede external obstacles from derailing your consistency. These shifts will ensure you don't get set back or regress by things like getting triggered by people and outside influences, getting overwhelmed with commitments, eating poorly at airports, or being tempted to overdo it at social events.

TRACY'S BREAKTHROUGH MOMENT

Lasting life changes often come because of breakthrough moments, and everyone's moment comes at a different time and in a different way. Tracy's breakthrough moment came on the later side, about four months into her six-month program. She was making good progress. She had learned the routine and the system. She was getting into a groove with her habits. She had lost most of the weight she wanted to lose and was feeling better about her body and her health.

But her initial success had made her comfortable. I could sense it when we talked on our coaching calls. She'd gotten some results, she looked better, she felt better. But her motivation was starting to wane. This caused her progress to plateau even though she hadn't yet reached her goal.

On one of our coaching calls over Zoom, she asked me, "Deekron, how do you keep going once you've already made some progress? I had a few social events lately and I can feel my old habits coming back. I mean, I know what to do, but I don't always feel like I want to do it. How do I keep it up?"

I paused and looked at her.

"Tracy," I said. "Why are you doing this?"

"What?" she asked, "What do you mean?"

"I mean, why are you in this program? Why did you sign up for this in the first place?"

She didn't have to think. "I wanted to feel good about myself again. I wanted to feel in control of my body and my health. I wanted to stop feeling like a failure."

"Okay," I said. "So, do you feel that way now? Do you feel in control? Do you feel good about yourself?"

She thought for a moment.

"Sort of? I mean, I feel better, and you've taught me so much about what to do that I do feel like I have some control, yes."

"It's up to you, Tracy," I said, "this is your decision. It comes down to how high you want to set that bar, and how badly do you want to reach that goal? If you're happy with your current results, then there's nothing more to do."

I paused.

"So, I'm going to ask you again: why are you doing this?"

She looked at me through the Zoom call, completely intent on the question. I could see the thought process happening on her face as she concentrated on how she was feeling, on what she wanted.

"Because I want to be the best possible version of myself."

"And are you the best possible version of yourself?"

Her whole demeanor changed as she gave her answer.

"Not yet."

CHAPTER 14

Mindset 101

"Survival is the thing. The mind will twist to survive. Anything can become normal."
—Harlan Coben

We're about to set the stage for something really important. Life-changing, in fact. You're about to learn how the mind works so you can conquer the three major mental challenges that arise when we try to transform our body in a lasting way.

You will make three shifts to overcome challenges in the "Mind" category that you learned about in Part II of the book.

To help you make these shifts, I'm going to explain to you how the mind is designed, and how its flaws and tendencies can continuously get in the way of your body and health goals. Only by transforming the mind can we transform the body in a lasting way.

Know that overcoming your mind's obstacles and its ingrained patterns will not be easy. After all, your mind has

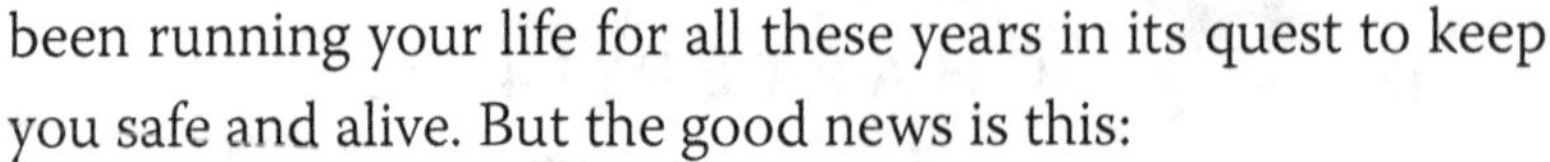

been running your life for all these years in its quest to keep you safe and alive. But the good news is this:

By gaining insights into how the mind works, you will become empowered to succeed at your body goals, as well as any goal that's important to you.

That's because the mind is at the center of everything—our work, our relationships, and our life. All of our outcomes come from our thoughts. How we show up in one area of our life is how we show up in all of them. As they say, "How we do one thing is how we do everything."

As vital as it is to learn about how our mind operates, most people never learn enough about this area. This leaves them stuck with the limitations of the mind, caught in the same patterns of stress, suffering, unhappiness, or unhealthiness.

And, unfortunately, most "mindset" content or advice is not going to save you.

WHY TYPICAL MINDSET ADVICE IS BULLSHIT

The word "mindset" gets thrown around these days; used very loosely by lots of people. There's no shortage of mindset podcasts, motivational YouTube videos, stoic quotes, or social media memes (#motivationmonday, anyone?). Most health & wellness influencers and coaches naively believe that they have expertise in this very complex area. They say things like, "You just need the right mindset!" or, "I can help you change your mindset!" Posts abound with superficial motivation tactics like pushing you to be "tougher" and not make excuses.

Unfortunately, it's (mostly) surface-level (and ineffective) advice.

Most folks who produce this content haven't done the deep transformational work and haven't developed the emotional intelligence required to transform a client's deep-seated beliefs, patterns, and habits.

Outside of words of encouragement, or regurgitating what they hear online, most health & fitness professionals are limited in their ability to impact a client's underlying mental and emotional make up in a way that's necessary for long-term behavior change.

Did hearing someone say, "mindset is everything," ever change your mindset?

Did reading a meme with "consistency is key" ever make you more consistent?

Did watching a "motivational" video ever keep you motivated for very long?

No?

Me neither.

In the best case, if you join a program, a well-meaning coach or professional may hold you "accountable" to help you with your body transformation. (By the way, this is another word that gets thrown around way too loosely, since all this usually means is temporarily losing weight, not a permanent transformation). While this accountability can help, it's short-lived. Once you stop working with said professional, the outside accountability disappears, and you're back to square one, with mostly the same thoughts, emotions, and patterns you had before you started working with them. Once they return, so do your old habits, and your old shape.

THE RIGHT WAY TO THINK ABOUT MINDSET

To truly transform our mindset, we need to dive below the surface. Your psychology and personality live in a deeper place—at the level of your emotions and in the subconscious mind. Like a SCUBA diver diving into deep waters to secure a treasure, this is the level we need to competently go to.

By going deeper, we better understand how our mind is wired, how the things we've been through influence how we see the world, and how our thought patterns help or hurt us.

I believe that proper mindset training is a special opportunity for true growth by gaining greater self-awareness, overcoming your past-based limiting beliefs, and transforming your entire way of being into someone who is more calm, powerful, loving, and free. Not to mention, more consistent with their habits and more skilled at overcoming obstacles.

The inner work I've done has made all the difference in how I show up in the world, and it gave me the courage to leave the corporate world, end toxic relationships, and follow my passion to help and empower others.

I firmly subscribe to the notion that transforming from the inside out is what's required for lasting change and that's where my team and I focus a good deal of our coaching efforts. Whether it's teaching you how to get and stay motivated or keeping you present to internal, fear-based patterns that seem to always trip you up—like perfectionism, procrastination, or self-criticism—my team and I passionately take on any mental blockers that could be derailing our clients from their goals.

Doing this type of inner work takes some courage and the right guidance, but when you embark on this journey, it changes your life forever. It paves the way for greater inner peace, confidence, happiness, and effectiveness in all areas of your life. It also paves the way for being more consistent with the habits needed to attain, and maintain, the body and health you desire.

My intention is that this book sparks your own journey towards transformation, enlightenment, and the life you've been craving.

Speaking of enlightenment, let's begin to uncover, at a very high level, how the mind is designed and how this design can get in the way of your body goals.

A HIGH-LEVEL OVERVIEW OF THE MIND

The mind has one primary mission: to ensure your survival.

A simple way to understand how your mind is designed is to think of these three P's.

- pain
- protection
- procrastination

PAIN (KEEPING YOU AWAY FROM IT)

Simply put, too much pain can lead to death. So, the mind is constantly monitoring to make sure that you're staying far away from anything painful. It's persistently using your five senses to scan the environment and analyze for threats to your well-being. As it does this, it moves you toward experiences that it perceives as safe (which you experience as enjoyable) and away from experiences it perceives as painful (which you experience as scary.)

For the things it can not grasp through sensory perception, the mind will try to understand through questioning. This has it constantly operating from a place of concern and worry, subconsciously asking existential questions like:

- "Am I OK?"
- "Am I safe?"
- "Am I at risk of pain?"
- "Am I accepted?"
- "Am I protected?"

This constant worry of the mind results in stress and negative internal states like anxiety and depression. This gives rise to our first mental challenge: emotional eating (i.e., stress eating).

PROTECTION (SEEKING IT FROM OTHERS)

In addition to keeping you safe from immediate threats and away from pain, the mind will also seek protection from those closest to you. As mentioned in Chapter 5, "Challenge #2: Limiting Beliefs", the mind is highly concerned with winning the love and approval of two groups of people: your parents and your tribe.

When we're born, we're helpless little babies who rely on the love and protection of our parents to survive. Without it, we die. Accordingly, a baby comes pre-programmed to instinctively seek out the love and protection of its parents. This is why children are always seeking the approval of parents, grandparents, or authority figures.

As we grow up, we need the protection of our tribe. If our tribe does not accept us and banishes us, other tribes or groups can hurt, abuse, or even kill us. It's this instinct that makes us highly concerned with fitting in, conforming to the group's rules, and keeping up with the Joneses.

To ensure your protection from others, there is one overarching question that the mind is concerned with the most.

"Am I good enough—to be loved (and protected)?"

This one question—about our self-worth—runs the show in the background of our lives.

If this question, "Am I good enough to be loved?" is not answered to the mind's satisfaction, and it fears that we indeed are not unconditionally accepted by those we subconsciously rely upon for protection, the mind begins to worry. It will subconsciously prompt us to overcompensate for any of our perceived shortcomings. In fact, this plays a big role in how our personalities are formed growing up.

When this overcompensation causes us to get burned out or overwhelmed or overly analytical, the first thing that usually takes the hit is our health habits.

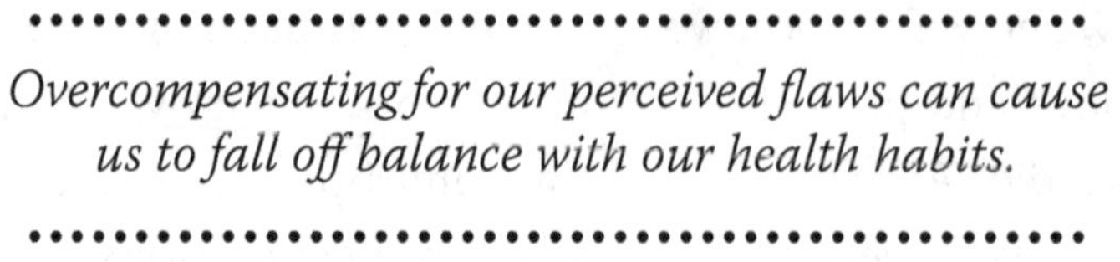

Overcompensating for our perceived flaws can cause us to fall off balance with our health habits.

This gives rise to our second mental challenge: limiting beliefs (and the overcompensation they cause).

PROCRASTINATION (AS A SURVIVAL STRATEGY, A.K.A. OUR "COMFORT ZONE")

I'm sure you've noticed that the mind is really good at putting things off. Procrastination is part of the mind's defense mechanism. If the mind perceives that something you think about doing can result in possible pain, it will come up with great reasons and clever excuses to justify delaying it.

Now there's a really big and important point you need to remember:

The mind can not differentiate between physical pain and emotional pain.

Hurt is hurt, whether it comes in the form of a punch in the nose or a pink slip in your face. It will do its best to avoid both.

Because the mind suffers when it doesn't feel successful or worthy (i.e., good enough to be loved), it will prevent us—very slyly—from doing things that can make us feel like a failure or to be rejected.

Asking someone out on a date, requesting a raise, pitching for a sale or speaking in public are all examples of situations that can result in feeling not good enough to be loved. It also applies to trying to lose weight again on a program because if we failed in the past, we dread feeling like a failure again.

In short, the mind will keep us away from anything that may cause pain or death. It will come up with clever reasons as to why it's better not to do something. Creative reasons to stop us from doing something can be along the lines of:

- Ask her out—"She probably has a boyfriend."
- Give that speech—"I'm too busy."
- Ask for the sale—"I don't want to come across as pushy."
- Try to lose weight—"I'll start next week."

Buying into these excuses is human nature. The problem is it leads to procrastination.

Procrastination is your comfort zone at work.

THE MAIN SOURCE OF MISSED WORKOUTS

You may not know this, but, subconsciously, the mind hates exercise. That's because any kind of exertion requires energy, and running out of energy can lead to death, so the mind's default mode is to resist exercise. That's still no excuse for skipping our workouts, but at least now we have an explanation for it!

Procrastination leads to a lack of action.

Lack of action leads to a lack of progress.

Lack of progress leads to a lack of motivation.

Lack of motivation keeps us stuck until we get frustrated or desperate for change; then we use willpower, which never lasts and we're back to procrastinating again.

This gives rise to our third mental challenge: wavering motivation (due to procrastination.)

A FINAL NOTE ABOUT THE MIND

Due to our core limiting belief that runs in the background of our lives, anytime we're reminded that we may not be good enough to be loved, say through a failure, rejection, comparison, criticism, or disappointment, these negative feelings can get triggered.

In turn, those negative feelings lead to negative thoughts, which lead to more negative feelings and more negative thoughts. This perpetuates a cycle of negative internal states that can lead to conditions like anxiety, depression, and impostor syndrome.

In fact, this is the root of much of our suffering.

The mind suffers. That's one of its modes.

Between constantly wondering if we're good enough to be loved, and looking out for potential threats and harm, it's no wonder then, that the majority of our thoughts are negative ones. In fact, scientists believe that 75% of our thoughts are negative thoughts.[34]

In short, the suffering our negative thoughts trigger can result in emotional eating, cause us to overcompensate and fall off track with our good habits, and dampen our motivation to eat well and exercise consistently.

The good news is this. In the pages that follow, you're going to learn how to prevent mental challenges from derailing your body and health, by learning how to master your emotions, rewire your limiting beliefs, and keep your motivation consistently high. All while reducing the mind's suffering and replacing it with greater peace and happiness.

These outcomes won't only change your body, they will totally elevate your life.

So, are you ready to start transforming your mind?

Master Your Emotions

1

Emotional Eating
Limiting Beliefs
Wavering Motivation

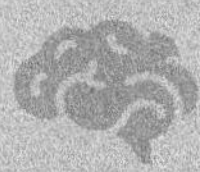

BODY

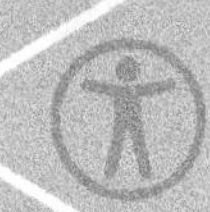

Slowing Metabolism
Changing Hormones
Injuries & Limitations

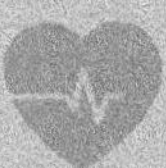

LIFE
High Stress
Limited Time
Travel & Social

CHAPTER 15

SHIFT #1: Master Your Emotions

"The greatest weapon against stress is our ability to choose one thought over another."
—William James

Mindset transformation loading . . .

Mastering your emotions is the first component of *The Nine Shifts*, and an essential part of your journey. As we learned in the last chapter, most people are unaware of why their mind causes suffering, and don't have strategies to manage these emotions. As a result, they rely on coping mechanisms like comfort foods, alcohol, or other substances to numb the pain. If this becomes habitual, it can hurt our body and our health.

To overcome this mental challenge, we need to make a key shift.

KEY SHIFT

Go from letting negative emotions affect your mood and habits to gaining greater self-awareness that leads to more internal peace and improves your ability to avoid bad habits.

Learning about how the mind works will give us greater clarity and power over our emotions.

DON'T BUY INTO THE SUFFERING OF THE MIND (OR THE MEANINGS IT MAKES)

Gym bros have a saying, "pain into power," which means take the pain you feel and channel it into your workout. While this is a healthier coping mechanism than, say, drinking or binge eating, I don't think this is quite enough. To me, it's more empowering to understand why you feel pain in the first place so you can transform it and stop it in its tracks.

Would you like to know why?

When we feel emotional pain, it's usually due to our interpretation of what's happening and what we make it "mean" about ourselves. For example, if I fail at enrolling someone into our transformation program, I can make that mean something about me: "It was my fault. I suck at this. I'm going to struggle and be a failure." This interpretation is one of many possible interpretations, but is one that could leave me frustrated and feeling emotional pain. As you now know, anything that reminds us of our inadequacies and causes us to feel "not good enough to be loved," will cause suffering in the mind.

The goal is not to suppress or avoid this pain, but to identify how the meaning the mind makes can cause us to suffer. In this way, we can choose a more empowering meaning and transform the agony into peace and calm.

When we become more present to the meanings the mind makes and how they can trigger emotional pain, stress, or suffering, we can avoid buying into them and letting them take over our mood and our habits.

Instead of just coping with the suffering, become wiser and more aware of what creates it in the first place—the meanings we make about ourselves.

This gives you the power to choose how you respond to your interpretations and your emotions, rather than just reacting to them. You get to the source and nip it in the bud. It's like the difference between cutting and weeding. If you only cut a weed you have to keep cutting it again and again every time it grows back. If you pull it out by the roots it never grows back.

From there, it becomes easier to stay grounded and consistent with everything we're up to, including limiting emotional eating so we can attain and maintain the body and health we're after.

We transform the mind, so that it allows us to transform the body.

Otherwise, the mind's default tendency to cause suffering can lead us to cope with these feelings through stress eating or to lose our balance and forgo our good habits.

THE APPROACH

To provide you with greater power over internal stress, The Emotional Mastery Plan in this chapter will take you through a three-step process that helps regulate negative emotions without relying on negative coping mechanisms.

First, it will teach you how to tell the difference between your mind's thoughts and the real you. This will provide greater peace and reduce negative emotions.

Second, you will come up with practical outlets for processing any pain that may arise, for whatever reason. This will allow you to quickly release pain and not let it throw you off for an extended period of time.

Third, you will come up with a list of healthy coping mechanisms, including better food and drink options, for when you need to withstand negative emotional states like anxiety, depression, self-loathing, etc. This way, what you choose to numb the pain with will have a small impact on your body and health.

To ensure negative emotions don't get the best of you, we need to empower you with strategies to keep you grounded and aware of how your mind could be trying to bring you down.

THE THREE-STEP EMOTIONAL MASTERY PROCESS

If you want to want to keep negative emotions and stress eating at bay, do this:

1. Distinguish between your thoughts and the real you (your essence)
2. Have healthy outlets for emotional pain
3. Choose better coping mechanisms

YOUR THOUGHTS VERSUS YOUR ESSENCE

Repeat after me:

"***I am not my thoughts.*** I have thoughts, but my thoughts are not who I am."

Repeat it again, and make sure you are saying it out loud. Transformation only happens through repetition. The more you read it and say it aloud, with *feeling*, the more your subconscious mind starts to believe it.

To gain power over the mind, and its tendency to suffer and keep us stuck, it's essential to understand the difference between who you truly are and the thoughts you're having (yes, even the ones you're having now as you're reading this book).

I describe who we truly are as our ***essence.***

Your essence has nothing to do with your identity, gender, religion, or your name. It's the "soul" part of having a mind, body, and soul. Your essence is not something you need to think about or describe in words. It's something you ***feel*** in your body. It speaks to you primarily through emotion, intuition, and hunches, not through thinking or words. It's the thing that lights up inside of you when you're with someone you love, do something you're proud of, or are dancing to your favorite song. It's the thing that is "moved" inside of us when we see an act of kindness and it's the hurt that we feel when we see another human suffering. Unlike our thoughts, our essence never comes and goes. It's always there. It's been there since the moment we were born and will be there until our last breath.

On the other hand, our thoughts mostly come from our mind. The mind analyzes, assesses, and tries to understand and make sense of the world. What's safe? What's threatening? Who's a friend? Who's an enemy? To ensure our safety, it's standing on guard to keep us protected. But all of this non-stop analysis doesn't allow our real essence to communicate with us. The mind tries to distract us and keep us in what feels safe, certain, tangible, and familiar. Certainty and familiarity are the mind's BFFs. Uncertainty and unfamiliarity are its enemies.

Author H.P. Lovecraft said, "The oldest and strongest emotion of mankind is fear, and the oldest and strongest kind of fear is fear of the unknown." That's because what is unknown, especially if we're in a dark alley or wild jungle, can kill us. By differentiating between your essence and your mind's thoughts you can begin to pick and choose what thoughts you listen to.

At one level, most of us know that some of our thoughts are completely off the wall and it's best not to listen to them. For example, we may feel like punching our boss in the face at times, but (luckily!) we know not to listen to that thought because we have another thought that reminds us that there are consequences to such impulsive (though tempting!) actions. Here, the mind is doing a good job of catching itself.

In other cases, we don't differentiate if the thought, and its corresponding feeling, is good for us or not. We just blindly go with it. For example, if we have a thought that says, "I'll just watch another episode of this series," even though it's already past midnight and staying up another hour will hurt our productivity the next day, we might just go with that thought, not noticing that the mind is leading us astray.

You may also get stuck trying to analyze your thoughts (overthinking, much?). If you rely on your thoughts for guidance or for making big decisions, it can sometimes feel like you're playing a game of ping pong in your head—overanalyzing, weighing pros and cons, evaluating and trying to figure out the best answer or solution.

The mind is not a place of peace,
nor is it a place of clarity.

In addition to certainty and familiarity, the mind's other BFF is the past. The mind doesn't know what's possible without proof. So, it relies on what happened in the past to predict the future. It decides what's possible in the future, based on what was possible in the past. If it's never been done before, the mind has no idea if it's possible, so it will ignore or try to avoid taking the risk. While some people are more risk averse than others, we certainly all have a risk tolerance and will shut down anything that we perceive may lead to loss or pain of some kind.

Needless to say, sticking only to what's familiar or known can limit us. It keeps us in the same patterns, doing the same things, working at the same job, following the same workout routine, and seeing the same people over and over. It may have seemed ridiculous when Bill Murray repeated the exact same day over and over in the (hilariously) satirical movie *Groundhog Day*, but for most of us, repeating the same cycle, as if we were stuck on a hamster wheel, is not that far from our reality.

The way to get out of this trap is to start differentiating between your mind's thoughts and your true essence.

The peace and clarity you seek exist on the other side of the mind's persistent thinking. When you can pull back and observe what the mind is doing, with its constant thoughts and analysis, you can begin to bring your awareness into your body—where your real essence lives. There's nothing but calm and peace there. Your thoughts come from your mind. They live "upstairs." Your essence speaks to you through emotion. It lives "downstairs," in your body.

In the book, *Don't Believe Everything You Think,*[35] author Joseph Nguyen advises us to learn the difference between a real thought and the thinking we do around that thought. This is a good way to discern our mind's thinking from your actual essence trying to speak to you.

Thinking About It versus Feeling about It

Another way to tell the difference between you and your mind's thinking is to feel. My cousin, Emanuela (who I consider a soul sister and someone who is just as committed to growth as I am), taught me to get out of my head and ***feel*** into my body whenever I have an important decision to make. It works for anything—business decisions, relationship matters, home buying . . . even ordering brunch; you name it!

It's often referred to as a "gut feeling" or "your higher self." From a metaphysical perspective, your essence (which speaks to you through your body) is your soul and your soul is part of the universe. As such, it's connected to all of the wisdom in the universe. This is where your intuitive abilities stem from. To tap into your intuition and have the infinite wisdom of the universe guide you, calm the mind, and feel into your body. Give the mind a break and let your intuition take over.

This requires letting go and trusting, which is not always easy. It's hard for the mind to trust when it doesn't know where a decision will lead you. It's even harder to trust if you've been hurt or have experienced loss in the past. But quiet the mind and feel into your intuition.

You'll know you're doing it right when you become the observer of your thoughts.

Interact with your thoughts like a cinema goer watching a movie, instead of being the actor in the movie.

Learning to differentiate between your thoughts and yourself will start to alleviate the suffering and the negative feelings and the internal stress you've been battling for so long. When you realize that there's nothing to battle, and your survival is ensured, you become master of the mind's constant chatter. You will hurt less, it won't last as long, and you won't have to rely on substances just to get through the day.

You—the real you—will emerge.

Addressing the inside first will allow you to properly address the outside.

Transforming the mind allows the work of transforming the body to begin.

HEALTHY OUTLETS TO EASE EMOTIONAL PAIN

Even with the tools above to reduce pain and suffering, sometimes those emotions are going to win. So, it's important to have a healthy outlet or a go-to routine that helps you get out of the suffering of the mind, and moves your attention and energy into your heart and into your body.

One thing you can do when you feel emotional pain is to move your body. Movement is the best medicine there is, and it's practical. In fact, they say that exercise is the greatest antidepressant ever invented. In one Australian study, a regular exercise regimen was shown to be 150% more effective at treating depression than subjects who took antidepressants.[36]

But it doesn't have to be formal exercise. It can be anything—a short walk, a few jumping jacks, chasing your dog or cat, or dancing.

Tony Robbins says "Motion creates emotion." Meaning that movement creates positive feelings. So just move, often. Move when you're down, move when you're happy, move as much as you can. Not only does your body need it, your mind needs it too.

Want to do one even better? Move to music! Your favorite

Motion Traxx (If you'd like to check it out, here's the link. Or scan the QR code to download and get five free sessions when you sign up; no credit card required. **www.motiontraxx.com**

tunes have the power to shift your emotions instantly. Music is so powerful, it's even used in healing traumas.[37]

The combination of movement and music is so close to my heart that, some years ago, I founded a tech startup that launched a fitness app called Motion Traxx, which syncs audio workouts by personal trainers to motivating beats to give people that extra push.

Besides moving, another thing you can do when you're anxious or down is to do something creative, like writing, drawing, painting, or playing an instrument. Creative pursuits get us out of our heads and connect us with our essence. There is creativity in all of us. When we pour our creativity into something positive, we also train the mind to be calm and we connect with our true essence.

CHOOSE BETTER COPING MECHANISMS FOR WHEN THEY'RE NEEDED

If the techniques above still don't work (sometimes they won't), and we need to numb the pain, it's best to proactively think about what your go-to coping mechanism will be versus just grabbing what's available. For instance, polishing off your kids' Oreos is probably not the best coping mechanism for your down days. Not only will your kids be annoyed if you finish their cookies (rightfully so!), but so will your digestive tract.

According to Charles Duhigg, author of *The Power of Habit*[38] a habit is made up of three parts: a trigger, a coping mechanism, and a reward. The trigger is often out of our control (a stressful day at work), and the reward is what we seek to deal with the negative emotions caused by the trigger (something that will make us feel good). But the coping mechanism is totally ***in*** our control. Making some smart substitutions when you feel stressed or depressed can go a long way towards minimizing their impact on your health and waistline, such as having seltzer water with a splash of juice instead of soda pop, some 70% dark chocolate instead of a pint of ice cream, or some chewing gum instead of a cigarette.

Along these lines, it also helps to not keep tempting items in the house. Do a cupboard cleanout and get rid of things like liquor, sweets, chips, soda pop, and other unhealthy items or vices you can reach for when in a distressed emotional state. It makes it harder to have junk when there's none of it around!

THE EMOTIONAL MASTERY PLAN

GUIDELINES

- Block off about 5–10 minutes to do this exercise.
- Grab a piece of paper, a pen, and find a quiet area.

- Start with your short meditation and answer the questions. There's no right or wrong answers, just write what comes to you without overanalyzing or trying to get it right.
- Above all, have fun with this! Make it an enjoyable part of your transformation journey.

There are worksheets available for each Action Plan that you can write on as you do the exercises. You can sign up to get them at: thenineshifts.com/downloads

PREP: GET GROUNDED AND GRATEFUL

Before doing any kind of mindset work, it's important to first get grounded and calm the mind. It's easy to do with this short, three-step gratitude meditation. Gratitude is one of the best ways to center yourself and release negative thoughts or emotions. Simply grab a pen and paper and a quiet moment and do the following.

Mini Meditation

- Close your eyes and take five, strong, deep breaths. (Brace your core as you exhale.)
- Keeping your eyes closed, think of things for which you feel blessed. (Family, friends, a roof over your head, a beloved pet, or similar.)
- With your pen and paper, write down everything you thought of and anything else that comes to mind. No limits.

That's it. Now you're in a grounded, centered place and ready to do the other exercises in this Emotional Mastery Plan.

STEP #1: DISTINGUISH YOUR MIND VERSUS THE REAL YOU

This pair of meditation exercises will help you observe different states so you can learn to recognize your mind's thoughts versus your essence.

Identifying When It's the Mind

With your pen and paper handy, in your quiet space, close your eyes and think about something or someone you really dislike or even hate. (Yes, even your ex if you'd like!) Or, if you have strong opinions about a particular topic (e.g., a political view, religious stance, or sports team), you can think about people that hold the opposite view as you do.

Keeping your eyes closed, focus on any of the sensations in your body. Where in your body is the negative emotion? Your head? Your chest? Notice everything you can.

Open your eyes and use your paper or journal to answer the following questions:

- How do you feel right now?
- What emotions are you present to?
- Where in your body are you feeling them?

Continue immediately to the next exercise.

Identifying When It's the Real You

Close your eyes again, but this time, think of something or someone you deeply love. You can even imagine yourself being in your happy place or doing something that brings you sheer joy. You can visualize spending precious time with someone you love, playing with a child, competing in sports, doing your favorite hobby or traveling to your favorite place.

Keeping your eyes closed, focus on any of the sensations in your body. Where in your body is the positive emotion? Your heart? Your gut? Notice everything you can.

Open your eyes and use your paper or journal to answer the following questions:

- How do you feel right now?
- What emotions are you feeling?
- Where in your body are you feeling them?

By observing both states, you now have a way to identify when it's your mind versus when it's the real you.

If you feel negative emotions, tight or tense in the body, stressed in the mind, analyzing, judging, etc., this is YOUR MIND doing the talking. The mind (i.e. the ego) judges and creates separation from others.

If you feel positive emotions, ease and energy in the body, enthusiasm in your mood, and you're free from any judgment or analysis, this is THE REAL YOU doing the talking. The real you creates connection and ease, and above all, it does not judge or have to be "right" about things.

STEP #2: BUILD HEALTHY OUTLETS

Now, we're going to brainstorm and choose some go-to outlets and strategies for when we feel emotional stress.

As I've said, a big one I always recommend is movement. Moving gets us out of our head and into our body. It can be any kind of movement you enjoy. A quick walk, bike ride, yoga, anything you like. If you don't have a lot of time, some jumping jacks, squats or pacing a bit can make a difference. If you can push past the emotion just enough to get yourself to exercise, it can be a powerful way to channel any stress you feel and shift into a powerful state, thanks to the endorphins you will feel. Other mechanisms that can soothe stress and shift you out of a negative state include:

- closing your eyes and taking three deep breaths
- thinking about someone you love
- focusing on something you love about yourself
- putting on your favorite song/station
- doing something creative like writing or painting
- giving gratitude

Your turn! On your paper or in your journal, brainstorm as many things as you can think of that feel good, make you happy, or are a form of movement you enjoy.

Choose one or two to be your "go-to" strategies for when stress or negative emotions hit and write them down. You might even want to put them on sticky notes or on your desktop or phone background so you can remember them in the moment.

Now, practice using them when you feel stressed, afraid, angry or have other negative emotions!

STEP #3: CHOOSE BETTER COPING MECHANISMS

Even if we use our healthy outlets to shift into a positive state, our emotions can sometimes still get the best of us. For those times, you will want to have healthy coping mechanisms at the ready. If you tend to reach for junk food when you're stressed, then having decided ahead of time on a healthier option (that you still enjoy) will make it easier to make healthy choices in the moment.

For example, here are some of my favorite healthy snack substitutes:

- air popped chips (instead of fried potato chips)
- carrot sticks with hummus (instead of corn chips)
- yogurt and nuts (instead of pizza)
- 70% dark chocolate (instead of milk chocolate)
- fruits like strawberries (instead of cookies)
- flavor-infused sparkling water (instead of soda pop)

Now, with your pen and paper or journal, take a few minutes and brainstorm answers to these questions:

1. What are the foods you tend to reach for when you are stressed or upset?
2. What are all the healthy food, snack and drink options you really love?
3. What could be some of your go-to substitutes for when you need to cope with negative emotions?

Choose a few to add to this week's shopping list, and practice choosing the healthier option you've selected for yourself.

Pro Tip: Don't buy the fatty, salty, sugary treats that you tend to trip over, and give away any of them that are left in the house!

Amazing work! You just fully completed this chapter.

Keep going and keep your transformation moving forward!

Master Your
Emotions

Rewire Limiting
Beliefs

1

2

MIND
Emotional Eating
Limiting Beliefs
Wavering Motivation

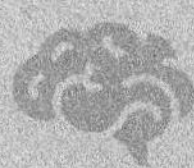

BODY
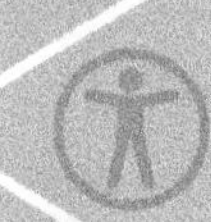
Slowing Metabolism
Changing Hormones
Injuries & Limitations

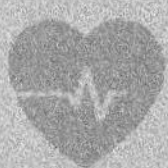

LIFE
High Stress
Limited Time
Travel & Social

CHAPTER 16

SHIFT #2: Rewire Limiting Beliefs

"Care for your psyche . . . know thyself, for once we know ourselves, we may learn how to care for ourselves."
—Socrates

Alright, now we're going to do something a little different.

Since you've done such a great job to this point in the book, I'm going to share a really cool story with you about my client Faith; she used to struggle mightily with perfectionism and yo-yoing weight. By hearing about how we helped her revisit her childhood years to transform her limiting beliefs and identity, you'll learn what it takes to overcome any limiting beliefs and overcompensations that are holding you back.

Remember, overcompensation, by pulling at our energy, time, and attention, can result in leaving our health habits by the wayside and cause us to lose our balance and be inconsistent. To conquer this challenge, this chapter will empower you to make the following key shift:

KEY SHIFT

Go from operating blindly inside of a fear-based identity that makes you overcompensate and procrastinate doing your health habits, to uncovering your core limiting belief and identity, so you can transform them and free yourself to take action consistently.

By going through this chapter and the Belief Rewiring Plan you will learn what it takes to shift into a new, more empowering identity that will provide you freedom from limitations. It will allow you to go easier on yourself, speak up and express yourself, and to create the boundaries—within yourself and with others—so you can consistently be in action and maintain the habits that will keep your metabolism elevated, your body lean, and your health optimal.

It's not easy or overnight, but if you're willing to do the work and go beyond surface-level advice and social media memes to transform the right way, you will begin to reinvent yourself at the deepest level of who you are. Your beliefs will change. How you see yourself will change, you will take on a more empowering story about your self-worth, you will minimize impostor syndrome, and you will step into a more empowered version of yourself. Furthermore, you will make peace with what you've been through and begin to heal the wounds of that scared little person who's been suppressed inside of you for all these years, just trying to survive.

If you get this right, it will be the most profound shift you've ever experienced in your life. I know it was for me. It is for my clients, too.

To help clients begin to heal their past, we take them through a powerful, proprietary mindset coaching session called Rewind & Reframe™. It's designed to take you back in time and uncover your core limiting belief (the one that started when you were a child), wipe the slate clean, and come up with a more empowering belief and identity to guide your life and your actions.

Clients that have been through one of my Rewind & Reframe™ sessions have had massive breakthroughs. It's helped them to gain greater self-awareness, and to see, for the first time in decades, how their past-based, childhood-derived, fear-based beliefs are still running the show and limiting them. Once they transform these ingrained beliefs and embrace a more empowering identity, they break free from limitations, make better decisions, and excel in the areas in which they were being held back, including in their career, relationships, and their health.

One amazing woman who's had a life-changing breakthrough in self-awareness and personal power is my client, Faith.

HOW FAITH "THE PERFECTIONIST" REWIRED HER LIMITING BELIEFS TO TRANSFORM HER MIND, BODY, AND LIFE FOR GOOD

My client, Faith, is a seasoned marketing executive for a Fortune 1000 manufacturing company in the Midwest. Any time her stress and workload got too high, she'd stop doing her health habits.

As a result, her weight would fluctuate in lock-step with her stress levels. This situation frustrated her and she was desperate for a solution. She knew that unless she got to the bottom of what was causing her to drop off her habits every time stress or work got intense, she would be at the mercy of those factors for the rest of her life.

Anytime we feel stuck in an area, there most likely is a limiting belief holding us back.

To help Faith uncover what could be stopping her, I took her through my Rewind & Reframe™ breakthrough session I describe above.

During Faith's session, I learned that her family moved around a lot when she was young, which made it hard to have close friends. Her parents also fought a lot. This caused Faith to begin questioning whether their fighting was because of her and whether or not they loved her. She told me that, at one point, questioning their love for her, she slipped a note under their door, asking them "Do you love me? Please check the box below: Yes or No."

As a child, she (incorrectly) interpreted that the fighting between her parents was happening because of her and that she had no place in that family.

Faith's limiting belief was "I don't belong."

To overcompensate for this perceived shortcoming, Faith subconsciously decided to try to win the acceptance of her parents by studying harder in order to get good grades. She certainly didn't want to be the reason for their fighting any longer. This became her survival strategy.

She also started taking on all kinds of extra curricular activities that she knew would please her parents. She was unconsciously doing her best to be the perfect child in order to win their love.

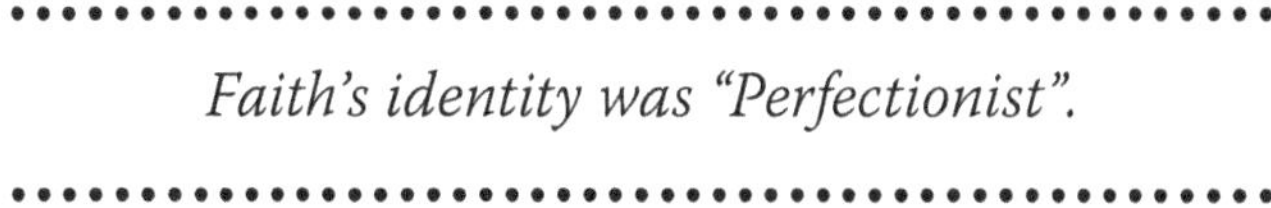

These findings are not uncommon. For most perfectionists, the need to please their parents is the seed of their perfectionism. The fear of not being accepted makes them cover their fear by looking, acting, and being perfect. But deep down they're scared. I've heard my friend, Petra Kolber, author of the *Perfection Detox*[39] use this clever metaphor on her podcast: "Perfectionism is fear dressed up in nice shoes."

Now, observe how our early traumas stay with us throughout our lives, unless we transform them . . .

As an adult, Faith spent her life working harder and harder, especially during times when she'd start at a new job. Like she did with her parents, Faith would be eager to win the acceptance of her new superiors and feel like she "belongs." Her survival strategy of winning people over through her accomplishments (i.e., just like getting good grades to please her parents) and her identity of being a perfectionist would cause her to take on more and more work. She would even take on outside obligations, like getting a master's degree.

When all the work she'd take on would start feeling like it was too much, she'd get to the point of overwhelm, and the first thing she'd do is cut out her health habits. To compound the problem, she'd cope with the stress with comfort foods or snacks, and her mind would justify it by telling her that she "deserved it" for all of the hard work she was putting in. Not coincidentally, food was used as a reward by her parents when she was growing up.

As a result of this overcompensation-fueled overwhelm, which led to procrastinating on her health habits and turning to comfort foods, Faith's weight would start going up.

After seeing that her weight went up again during one of our weekly check-ins, Faith lamented, "With increasing workload at work and at school I got frustrated and gave up—typically happens when I'm tired and I'm used to rewarding myself with my favorite foods."

You can see how her weight would yo-yo every few months in her weight loss graph below.

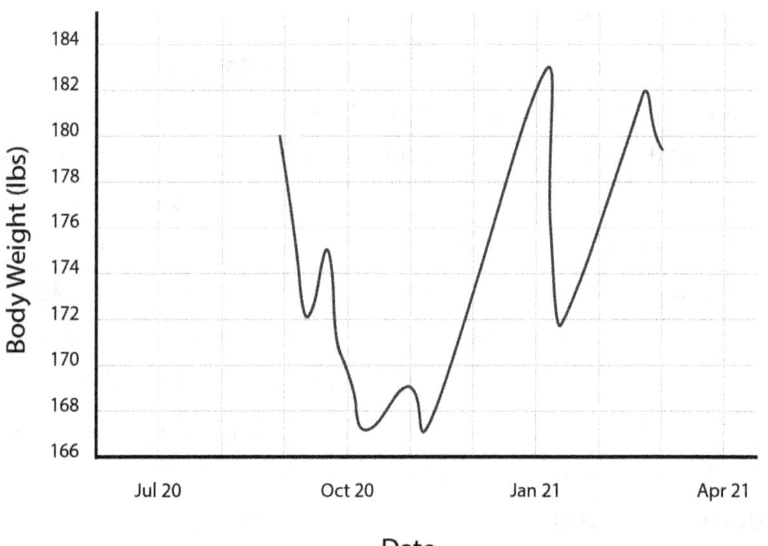

This imbalance would go on for a while. Being a perfectionist, she would wait until work would die down (it rarely did) to get back on track and would keep delaying until she could find the time to follow her program perfectly.

Waiting for the perfect time to restart her routine would result in weeks, sometimes months, of being sedentary and not eating well.

Consequently, she'd keep gaining body fat and her weight would climb up until she would get alarmed at how heavy she had gotten, and then try to "rebound" hard the other way, going to extremes of dieting and trying tough workouts that her 59-year old body couldn't handle for very long.

This "all-or-nothing," going to extremes approach is common for many high achievers.

You can see how Faith's early childhood trauma, though fairly minor, shifted how she saw herself and caused a limiting belief that affected how she operated in the world. The overcompensation of her survival strategy of working really hard just to pacify her core limiting belief ("I don't belong.") would derail her ability to keep her body in a good place.

Once her blindspots around her core limiting belief, survival strategy and identity were revealed, we were able to help her shift into a new, empowering story. In short, she took on the new belief of "I belong," and her new story is "I don't need to prove myself."

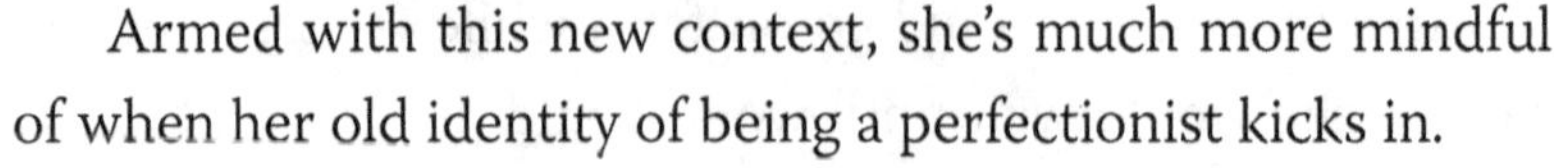

Armed with this new context, she's much more mindful of when her old identity of being a perfectionist kicks in.

This empowers her to resist the temptation of taking on more and more work just to prove herself.

She has also gained the courage to speak up and ask for resources (more staff, more budget, etc.) so that she doesn't take on the weight of the world and get overwhelmed again, risking her weight shooting up anew.

We also gave Faith a customized toolbox of habits and practices to use in order to keep the old limiting belief and survival strategy at bay, including the habit of taking imperfect actions, which you will learn about in Chapter 11, "Challenge #8: Limited Time."

Today, Faith holds her weight much more steady, rarely yo-yoing up and down like before. This is in spite of the fact her career and travel are still as demanding as ever. With her new level of self-awareness, she no longer needs to prove herself by overworking. This has given her more time, more calmness, and less stress in her life. It's also made her happier and more confident in her skin.

As you can see, Faith first had to transform in mind before she could see lasting change in her body. Greater self-awareness about how she's wired and rewriting her old, fear-based beliefs transformed how she thinks and behaves. She no longer sees her body transformation habits as something that needs to be done perfectly or that has to take a lot of time and effort. She fits it in when she can and allows herself to be less than perfect with them. Because of these changes, she is much more consistent with her habits than ever before. You can see the difference not only in her body but in the way she talks, moves and carries herself.

Faith says, "It feels different now."

And it shows.

"While the weight is coming off much more slowly than before—I am more confident that the weight will remain off as I continue to make good choices. Imperfect actions have really helped me with my weight, at work and in my personal life. Still writing my daily affirmation at the top of my to-do list everyday, and getting out and moving five times a week. Next step is to go ahead and invest in some bands and weights for my home due to the inconsistent availability of the gym."

THE APPROACH

In Chapter 5, "Challenge #2: Limiting Beliefs" we learned how the mind's need for protection from others makes it obsess over being "good enough" to win their acceptance. But when our initial, unresolved trauma makes us feel inadequate, we begin to chase validation by always having to be perfect, working too hard, acting too nice, or playing the victim.

To begin the process of properly rewiring your core limiting beliefs and identity and overcome these struggles, the Belief Rewiring Plan in this chapter will take you through a three-step, mini-transformation process.

First, it will help you explore your core limiting belief and recognize your identity. This will create much-needed self-awareness into your thought patterns.

	Perfectionist	People Pleaser
1. Determining Your Limiting Belief and Identity	"I need to be perfect and earn acceptance and validation through my achievements."	"I can't say no or people won't love me."
2. Take on a More Empowering Story	Accept being less than perfect; be OK and acknowledge progress each day instead of waiting until you arrive at your "destination" to feel happy.	Learn to courageously say "no" and speak up for what you need (including time for health habits and self-care).
3. Practice Being the New You	Take imperfect actions regularly; don't wait for the perfect time, perfect person, etc.	Tactfully communicate your needs and set proper, bold boundaries.

Second, it will help you make a mental shift to a new, more empowering story about yourself, one that is free from the past and aligned with your vision for your future self.

Third, you will come up with a simple ritual or affirmation that you can repeat daily in order to start practicing and transitioning into your new identity.

This process will enable you to overcompensate less, find more balance, and be more consistent. Just like my client Faith, who now takes on less work because her old belief of "I don't belong" no longer drives her to win approval through

Victim	Sacrificial Lamb
"Things happen ***to*** me. I'm trapped and powerless to change them."	"I can't trust others and need to do it all myself."
Remind yourself of gratitude and blessings. Know you're not at the mercy of your circumstances.	Start trusting and start asking for help. Practice patience and get people on your team.
Stay present to the times you accomplished something you're proud of or overcame difficulties. Remember that things happen ***for*** you, not to you.	Go over all the things you do each week and see which you can delegate. Ask for help regularly, clearly, and courageously.

perfection and hard work. She no longer allows herself to be all-or-nothing with her health habits any more. This means no more massive fluctuations in her weight.

Do this right and people around you will notice the new you (and your new body) emerging!

By implementing the strategies above, you will successfully shift your identity and avoid the overcompensations that have stopped you in the past from staying consistent with your health habits.

WE ALL HAVE TO START SOMEWHERE

The Belief Rewiring Plan coming up next will help you wipe the slate clean, and come up with a more empowering belief and identity to guide your life and your actions.

First, two important points.

I'm not a licensed therapist and this is not intended to be a replacement for seeking guidance from a certified mental health professional. (If you proceed with this exercise, you agree that you will do so at your own risk.)

That being said, I know enough, have learned enough, and had enough deep training around mindset and in my own transformation that I can help clients make these types of transformational mindset shifts. These shifts will give you more self-awareness and clarity so you can experience greater peace, and not let old patterns cause you to over-do or under-do your body transformation habits consistently.

Mindset can only shift so much from reading a book. It takes powerful introspection that's best led by a professional. This is what we do for our clients. (I'll share more about how we coach clients in this area along with ways to get help later in the book.) But don't worry, everyone's transformation journey starts somewhere, and this book is a great place to start.

Even starting to reflect on how you're wired can begin the process of change. The intention of this exercise is to get you to start exploring the limiting belief that is holding you back. Only by becoming aware of it, and releasing it every time it comes up, and replacing it with our new, more empowering identity, will we be free of the old one. Catch it when it comes up, thank it for trying to protect you, then release it so you can buy into your new, more empowering story and not do the overcompensating the old belief wants you to do in order to feel safe.

Remember that once you've taken on a new identity, it will not stick immediately. It will take a lot of practice to start living it and not letting the old fear-based self-belief come back. Transformation takes practice and repetition. A lot of it. And it never ends. You never "arrive."

I've been on a 20+ year transformation journey and it just keeps going. Every breakthrough you have will lead to a new breakdown. Every new breakdown you have will lead to another breakthrough. As the saying goes "New level, new devil."

Self-discovery is part of the game of life.

Otherwise, this journey would be boring, wouldn't it?

(You probably hate me by this point. But please don't hate me, because I have a life-changing gift for you: the keys to your new identity . . .)

THE BELIEF REWIRING PLAN

GUIDELINES:

- Time Required: 15–20 minutes
- What You Will Need: a pen, something to write on and a quiet area
- This will be an introspective exercise. You will be reflecting back on your life to unveil some important insights about yourself.
- In fact, you may find it hard to think that far back. If

so, that's OK. Just close your eyes and do your best.

- Start with the short meditation as described and answer the questions. There's no right or wrong answer, just write what comes to you without overanalyzing or trying to get it right.
- If you have trouble finding your limiting belief, you can ask someone to help you with the questions. As another option, you can request the help of a professional to guide you. I usually help my clients find their core limiting belief during their Rewind & Reframe™ session in under an hour.
- Your mind may resist visiting some of your perceived flaws. Acknowledge it but gauge if you're comfortable enough and can drum up the courage to "go there." Only by healing our past and making peace with it can we create a new future that is free from our old limitations.
- IMPORTANT: Make sure you are in a good mental state when you do this exercise because it may stir up old feelings and emotions.
- If you currently take psychotropic or mental health medications, or have been diagnosed with a mental health disorder, please consult with a mental health professional before doing this exercise.

STEPS:

- ☐ Mini-meditation
- ☐ Become aware of your core limiting belief and identity
- ☐ Come up with a more empowering story and identity
- ☐ Practice being the new you (and stay vigilant against the old you)

PREP: GET CLEAR AND CONNECT TO YOUR POWER

Like in the last chapter's action plan, we will start by clearing the mind and getting centered. You will also connect with the best version of yourself by reminding yourself why you're awesome.

a. Mini Meditation

- Close your eyes and take five strong, deep breaths
- Get present to anything going through your mind—thoughts, feelings, opinions, judgements, etc. Observe them but don't attach to them. Let them float away.

b. Connect With Your Awesomeness

- Keeping your eyes closed, think back to your proudest accomplishment.
- What was it?
- When was it?
- What kind of person did you have to be to make that happen?
- Write it down.

STEP #1: BECOME AWARE OF YOUR CORE LIMITING BELIEF AND IDENTITY

Step #1a: Your Core Limiting Belief

Think about the young version of you, around the time you were five years old.

What was your relationship like with those around you? Your parents? Your siblings? Your classmates? Reflect on this and write it out with as much detail as possible.

Did anyone make you feel unsafe or unworthy in any way?

Did you observe abuse or did you, yourself, experience abuse directly?

What do you recall about how they made you feel about your own self-worth? (For example: made me feel like my parents fighting was my fault, made me feel like I was going to get hurt, made me feel like I didn't belong, etc.)

Thinking back to these trying experiences and how they made you feel, how might you have—as a naive, scared child still learning about the world—incorrectly come to a conclusion that something was wrong with you? In what way did you feel like you weren't good enough or were inadequate? What did you say to yourself, about yourself and your own self-worth? What did you say about your ability to measure up, belong, and be loved by those around you? This is your core limiting belief.

Step #1b: Your Identity

During this time in your life how did you try to prove to yourself or others that there isn't anything wrong with you? Another way to think about it is to ask, how did you try to cover up the fact that something might be wrong or inadequate about you?

How did you try to survive this situation of not being good enough? How did you try to cover up for being "less than?" How did you try to fit in or belong? This is your survival strategy.

How did you try to win the acceptance of others, given that there might be something wrong with you? How did you try to overcompensate for the limitation of your core limiting belief? Examples include: by getting good grades, being nice, never disobeying, always listening to your parents, not asking for much, or staying quiet and out of trouble.

In what ways do you feel you may still overcompensate now? Look for tendencies that you feel are just part of your personality. Examples include: being too nice, having a fear of saying no or setting boundaries, always trying to look or act a certain way, not giving yourself permission to fail, never asking for help and trying to do it all yourself, staying in toxic relationships to feel needed, or never being satisfied with your accomplishments, possessions, or status.

What identity has this led to? The four major ones are: The Perfectionist, The People Pleaser, The Victim, and The Sacrificial Lamb; or maybe you are a blend of more than one, or perhaps a different one altogether; write down one that feels right to you.

STEP #2: COME UP WITH A MORE EMPOWERING STORY AND IDENTITY

Thinking about how your experiences created a core limiting belief about your self-worth, which wasn't true, and how it shaped your identity, what is the opposite of that identity? If your identity is one of The Perfectionist, the opposite might be something like forgiving, content, accepting, patient, or trusting.

Think about what life is like for you if you were to reach your highest potential, meet all your goals and aspirations in the areas of health, wealth, love, and family. Visualize yourself in the future and look back from there. Then, ask yourself: "Who did they (you) have to be to get there?" Examples: courageous, patient, forgiving, self-expressed, healthy, disciplined, or consistent.

What is a new identity that would make you feel excited to take on? Even if it feels surreal or unrealistic, write down what comes to mind. This can be the opposite of the old identity like you wrote down before, or if something else comes to mind that would be exciting (e.g., strong, healthy, vibrant, or magnetic) add it here.

How would this new identity make you feel?

STEP #3: PRACTICE BEING THE NEW YOU (AND STAY VIGILANT AGAINST THE OLD YOU)

If we do nothing to establish our new identity, our old identity will be there waiting to pounce. It's already the mind's default view of you and it will fight to keep you there because the mind will protect everything that it associates with you, including how you see yourself and your identity. To establish your new identity, you have to take actions that prove to the mind you actually are this new person.

One way to greatly improve your chances of becoming this new person who is no longer encumbered by their past fears is to literally declare your new identity every day. The perfect time to do this is first thing in the morning because your conscious mind gets distracted by work and life.

Say your new identity and internalize it through strong emotions. Really feel it! The stronger the emotion, the deeper the neural connection it builds.

Better yet, write it out, declare it to yourself in the mirror, or say it to others.

Doing this daily, over and over, and you will start to notice a shift in your thoughts and your actions. You'll start acting in new, more empowering ways.

Old parts of your personality will start to melt away and be replaced with new traits that weren't there before, for example, patience, forgiveness, self-love, and courage.

If you truly did the exercise, I want to say great job! This is not easy work. It takes focus and courage. But it's the price for the life you truly want.

You'll be happy to know that your transformation is well on its way.

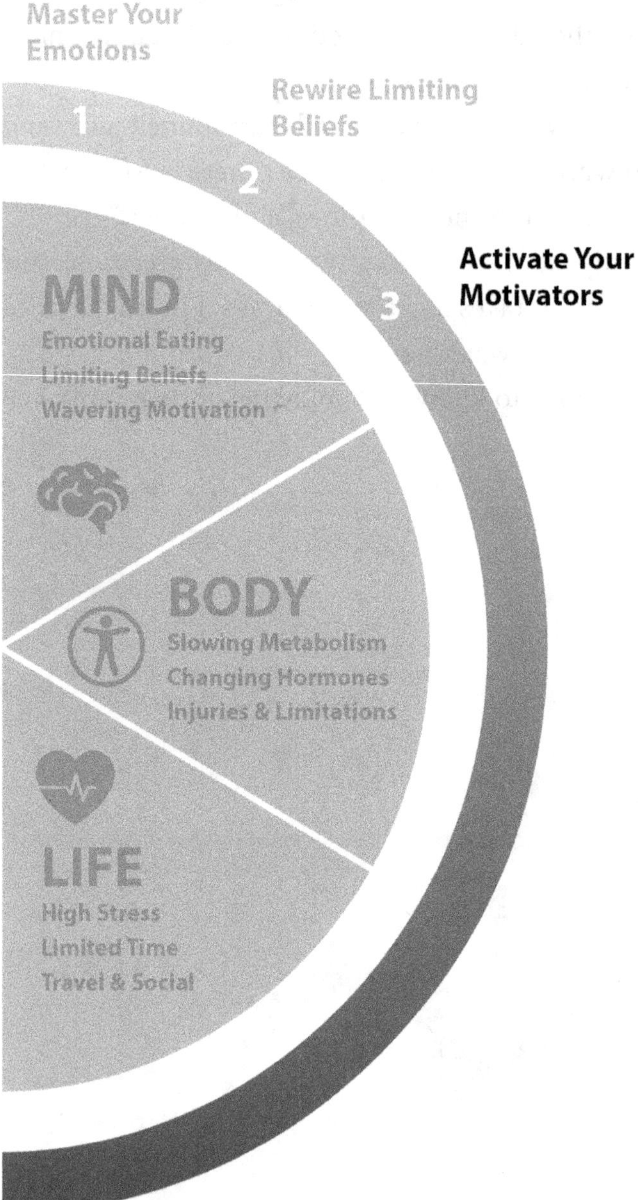

Master Your Emotions

1

Rewire Limiting Beliefs

2

Activate Your Motivators

3

MIND
Emotional Eating
Limiting Beliefs
Wavering Motivation

BODY
Slowing Metabolism
Changing Hormones
Injuries & Limitations

LIFE
High Stress
Limited Time
Travel & Social

CHAPTER 17

SHIFT #3: Activate Your Motivators

"You have power over your mind—not outside events. Realize this, and you will find strength."
—Marcus Aurelius

The third component of aligning your mind to achieve long-term success in your body is learning how to stay motivated consistently.

We've learned that the mind's comfort zone is a defense mechanism that loves to cause procrastination, which kills motivation. We also learned that most people misunderstand how motivation works, and end up believing myths and making mistakes, such as waiting to feel motivated before taking action. These missteps lead to inconsistency in their motivation level, their habits, and the state of their body.

To conquer this challenge, here is the key shift you will make:

KEY SHIFT

Go from waiting to feel motivated before taking action, relying solely on willpower, and making inconsistent progress, to taking simple actions even when not feeling motivated, tapping into inspiration for motivation, and ensuring you consistently see progress in your body transformation.

Making this shift will reduce the constant "starting, stopping, and starting over" that plagues many folks who struggle with their body.

THE APPROACH

The main objective with this shift is to overcome the resistance and reluctance that can keep us stuck and create extreme fluctuations in motivation, separated by long periods of waiting. Instead, we want to experience smaller fluctuations in motivation and more consistency in both our actions and our motivation level.

To stay motivated consistently, we want to shift out of vacillating between the two extremes of waiting and willpower, and shift into taking small, consistent actions in spite of any internal or external obstacles.

The Motivation Activation Plan is designed to ensure that you take action ongoingly, and those actions need to lead to results. Otherwise, we will have tried hard for nothing and this will deflate us and make us want to throw in the towel. If you want to keep your motivation high consistently, follow the three principles below.

LEVERAGE ONGOING EMPOWERMENT INSTEAD OF RELYING ON WILLPOWER

As we saw in Chapter 7, "Challenge #3: Wavering Motivation," most people go through extreme peaks and valleys of motivation. They'll push hard, often using willpower, when they feel eager—or even desperate—to make a change. For instance, after eating mindlessly for weeks and gaining weight during the holidays (i.e., the New Year's resolution setters).

Then, they'll get hit with stress, boredom, or life challenges, causing them to fall off their habits—partially or completely. This kills their progress, and along with it, their motivation. They struggle and stay in the "cycle of stuck" for a while until a triggering event happens (i.e., shocked at how they look in a photo, feeling dejected after receiving a critical

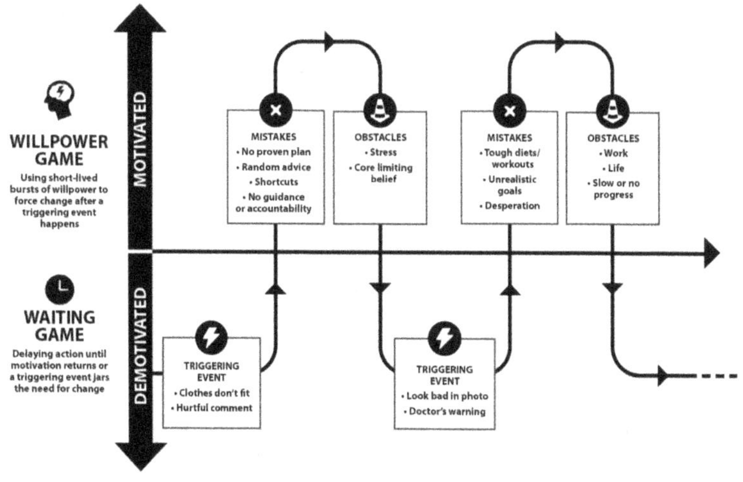

remark about their appearance, or getting a scary lab result on their annual check up). They resort to willpower again to start making changes. Their weight also yo-yo's up and down in lock step with these peaks and valleys in their motivation level.

This key shift, Active Your Motivators, will allow you to go from these extreme, roller-coaster like swings in motivation to a smoother, more controlled and more consistent level of motivation, like in the diagram below. This consistency will help you maintain your body where you want it over the long run.

Instead of relying on finite willpower to try to force your way to your goal, you will tap into ongoing empowerment to keep your motivation high.

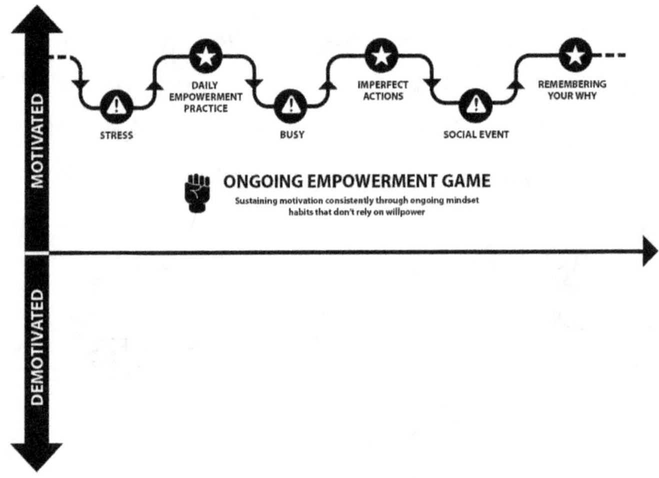

As you can see from the diagram, empowerment practices done regularly never allow your motivation level to drop too far. Ongoing empowerment allows you to "catch" motivation levels as soon as they drop and nudge them back up by doing something that's quick and easy, like a daily mindset habit or taking an imperfect action.

This makes it easy to sustain your motivation without a ton of effort, just like with our plane analogy that's cruising along at 30,000 feet versus the one that has to land and take off again.

ENSURE YOU'RE MAKING CONSISTENT PROGRESS

Remember, motivation is not a feeling you wait for, but an outcome of seeing progress. To stay motivated, we have to work the Motivation Loop properly.

The Motivation Loops diagram reminds us that to keep motivation going, the key is to take action, even when we

MOTIVATION LOOP

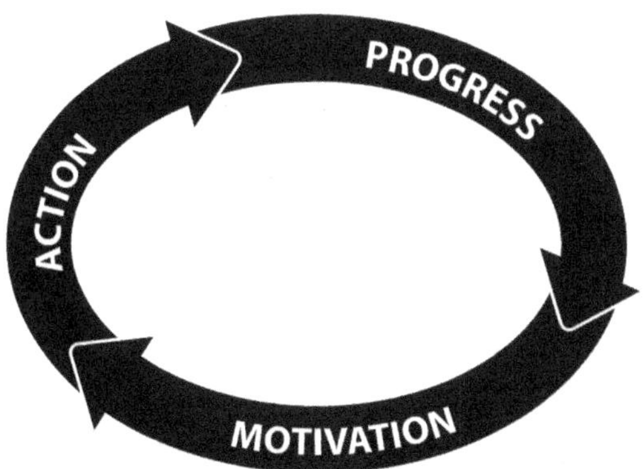

don't feel like it, without relying on willpower, while also ensuring that our actions lead to progress.

Sounds hard, but it's not.

To ensure consistent progress, we have to manage what I call the "4 E's of Consistency":

- **Environment**—Make sure that the people and structures around us ensure our success.
- **Enjoyment**—Make sure the process is fun; this prevents resistance or the need to use willpower.
- **Emotions**—Make sure stress or negative emotions don't kill our motivation.
- **Externals**—Manage obstacles from work and life from setting us back.

The exercises in the Motivation Activation Plan will ensure these consistency factors are managed. Additionally, the strategies you'll be learning throughout *The Nine Shifts* framework ensure that these four aspects of consistency are covered.

DON'T MAKE YOUR HABITS "OPTIONAL" (A.K.A. MY DAD'S LIFE ADVICE)

This one mental shift is very powerful, so please lean in and listen up. I want this one to really sink in—especially if you've ever struggled with motivation around your body transformation goals.

It's based on a lesson my dad taught me at a very young age. This lesson empowered me to not only achieve my body and health goals, but also to succeed at big life aspirations.

This key life lesson that my dad taught me was:

When it comes to doing things that are important, you don't give yourself an option. You do them.

This philosophy ties in perfectly to the mindset shifts you've been learning in *The Nine Shifts*:

- You do them because that's who you are (identity).
- You do them because that's what you believe in (your why).
- You do them even when you don't feel like it (the mind's comfort zone).
- You do them even when you think you can't (limiting beliefs).
- You do them even when it's hard (motivation).

When we don't give ourselves the option to not do something, we don't allow the mind's limiting beliefs, resistance, comfort zone, or excuses to win. Another way I like to frame it for my clients is to tell them to "not make the obstacle bigger than you." (Do the thing, despite the obstacle.)

The mind frame my dad taught me of "don't make it optional" is what's made the biggest difference in the things I've accomplished in my life.

This includes graduating from a premier Business School (The Ross School of Business at the University of Michigan), to working for global consulting firms, to securing a $200,000 sponsorship from a national advertiser (Gatorade) for my relatively unknown fitness podcast, to having my Motion Traxx fitness app featured by Apple for a year, and even to writing this book for a second time (after writing it once, scrapping it, and starting all over to produce something much, much better).

I don't share these things to brag but to share a bit more about myself and prove that we can accomplish big things when we don't make our important goals optional.

Now, I will admit that doing things "no matter what" sometimes means relying on your own internal fortitude, discipline, and willpower. Don't get me wrong. Developing those traits is very valuable. Indeed, they even get stronger the more you use them. So, in some cases using willpower to stay in action and get your habits done can be beneficial.

At the same time, trying to use willpower to always get in action is not a sustainable long term strategy for most people. Case in point: at the end of a long, stressful day at work, there is usually little willpower left over to endure a diet or do a tough workout.

Instead of willpower, connecting with a deeper, more meaningful "why" is a much better source for motivation and consistency.

In the fitness motivation book, *No Sweat,*[40] author Dr. Michelle Segar, Professor at The University of Michigan (my alma mater!) says, "The right whys motivate us because they are relevant to our daily lives and personally meaningful."

So, get clear on your "why" for achieving your goal, and make it meaningful. The more meaningful it is, the more it will motivate you to stick it out and find ways to reach your goals, even when things get tough. Jim Rohn taught us, "If the why is powerful, the how is easy."

I mean, no one climbs Mount Everest and risks their life simply because they're bored or feel like taking some cool photos. There has to be something deeper and more meaningful there.

Whether you use willpower or not to get your habits done, this philosophy of don't make your meaningful goals optional will make the difference between staying in action consistently and having the body, health, and life you desire, or failing to look, feel, and perform your best and (ultimately) setting yourself up for pain or regret.

So stay present to why it matters and don't give yourself the option to not do it. This is one of the greatest sources of motivation you'll ever tap into.

THE MOTIVATION ACTIVATION PLAN

GUIDELINES:

- Time Required: 10–15 minutes
- What You Will Need: A pen, something to write on, and a quiet area
- Start with the short meditation as described and then answer the questions. There's no right or wrong answer, just write what comes to you without overanalyzing or trying to get it right.
- Unlike the action plan that came before this one (for Belief Rewiring), which required deep introspection this action plan will be enjoyable and light.
- So, have fun with it and let's start mastering motivation once and for all!

STEPS:

- ☐ Mini-meditation
- ☐ Make a list of imperfect actions you can take
- ☐ Focus on fun
- ☐ Come up with an inspiring "InPowerment Word" (stay present to it)

PREP: GET CENTERED AND INSPIRED

As mentioned, before doing any kind of mindset work, it's important to first get centered and calm the mind. We'll start with a short, easy meditation in order to release any thoughts or emotions that might be present. Then, you will answer some questions that will improve your ability to keep motivation high consistently.

Mini Meditation

- Close your eyes and take five strong, deep breaths.
- Keeping your eyes closed, visualize yourself in the future, having accomplished your most important goals and attained your desire.
- Connect to that feeling, taking five more deep breaths.
- Write down why your goals inspire you. Write down what reaching your goals provides for you, and those around you.

That's it. Now you're in a grounded, centered place and ready to do the other exercises.

STEP #1: MAKE A LIST OF IMPERFECT ACTIONS YOU CAN TAKE

This step will help you stop waiting and help you take some kind of action, even when you don't feel like it.

This question will be fun and will encourage you to use some creativity.

What we're looking for here is a list of around five, go-to imperfect actions you can take when motivation is low or when thinking about a formal workout creates resistance in your mind. Simple actions that will create extra movement and calorie burn, that you can fit in easily into your day without much time, thought, or motivation required.

Examples include: taking the stairs instead of the elevator, parking on the far end of the parking lot to get extra steps in, taking a 10-minute brisk walk after dinner, doing twenty squats while watching TV, or doing a dozen push ups or jumping jacks before hopping in the shower.

If you like the ones above, feel free to use them. You can also come up with your own. Get creative!

STEP #2: FOCUS ON FUN

Remember that the mind, which is always worried about survival and what other people think, can sometimes be a heavy and dark place. If the journey is not enjoyable, we'll most likely quit. So, be sure to keep things light and fun.

Think about some ways to add fun to your routine.

Some examples include: going to a fitness class you really enjoy, rewarding yourself (smartly) after a tough workout or a consistent week, exercising with a friend that makes you happy, buying yourself some new workout clothes that'll feel good when you put them on, setting a goal to look great for a special event like a vacation, wedding, or reunion.

What are some ways you can make this journey more fun? Write them down now!

STEP #3: COME UP WITH AN INSPIRING "INPOWERMENT WORD"

This action will help you avoid having to rely on finite willpower and will keep you motivated consistently by tapping into inspiration, which is endless because it comes from your infinite essence.

To give my clients a simple tool to keep their mind focused and inspired, I help them come up with what I call an

InPowerment Word™. To ensure that it inspires you, your InPowerment Word has to be connected to something that is meaningful to you; it's kind of like your why or your purpose for your body transformation journey.

Here's how to find it:

- Close your eyes, take three deep breaths, and ask yourself "***Why*** is being my fittest and healthiest important to me?"
- The more meaningful your answer, the better.
- My clients usually respond with answers such as: "To be around to see my grandkids graduate," (longevity), "So I can be my best," (success), "So I can age well," (freedom).
- Come up with a list of about 5–10 meaningful reasons for being your healthiest and fittest and write them down. Boil each reason down to one word like I did above and write them down.
- Circle the one word that speaks to you the most. You can always change it later but for now, choose only one. That's your InPowerment Word!

Write it on a few sticky notes and paste them up around the house. Seeing them often will remind you of it and keep your mind focused on it over and over. Remember, transformation happens through REPETITION. To motivate and inspire yourself daily, recite your InPowerment Word every morning during your morning routine.

Amazing work! You just fully completed this chapter and are well on your way to sustaining your motivation consistently for life.

CHAPTER 18

Metabolism 101

"Everybody needs a hug. It changes your metabolism."
—Leo Buscaglia

Congratulations are in order, young Jedi. By immersing yourself in the last section, Mindset, you've taken an "inside-out" approach and have ensured that the mental challenges of emotional eating, limiting beliefs, and wavering motivation do not get in the way of your body and health goals. (Bravo!) Unlike most people who dive head-first into the latest fad diet or exercise routine, you've given yourself the best chance of staying consistent with the habits that will transform your body and ***keep you*** lean, healthy, and confident.

So, what exactly are those habits?

Well, that's the topic of this next section.

HOW THIS PART OF THE BOOK HELPS TRANSFORM YOUR BODY

The Metabolism part of the *Nine Shifts* body transformation framework will guide you to make three key shifts that will elevate your metabolism and make your body optimal:

1. Train For Strength
2. Optimize Your Nutrition
3. Enhance Your Sleep

These three shifts will empower you to overcome the challenges brought on by the body itself: slowing metabolism, changing hormones, and injuries & limitations.

By making these three shifts, we will reverse these age-related obstacles and improve all aspects of the body, including reducing body fat levels, increasing strength, stabilizing energy, reducing aches and pains, enhancing longevity, improving performance, and more. By creating—and maintaining—these changes in the body, you will enjoy greater confidence, peace of mind around your health, and a greater quality of life.

The three chapters that follow will share proven, science-based strategies and steps for shedding fat and adding muscle safely and naturally after the age of forty. You will learn how to properly execute your workouts to build strength and burn maximum fat.

You will also learn how to structure your meals in a way that will optimize your hormones to keep you lean, healthy, and energized throughout your day. In addition, you will learn how to enhance your sleep and recovery, a highly underrated aspect of the body transformation journey.

All of these three factors—training, nutrition, and sleep—will synergistically work together to help you transform your body by keeping your metabolism high, which, as you are about to see, is the real key for achieving the body, health, and energy you're after.

Don't be surprised if, by implementing these three shifts correctly, you start looking and feeling younger and people notice a new pep in your step!

A WORD TO THE WISE

One big reason people fail at transforming their body is because they're impatient. Due to a lack of time or desperation to fix themselves, they come to me with a "Just tell me what to do" attitude.

As someone who can be pretty impatient myself, I totally get it.

While I love "cutting to the chase" and just being told what to do, if we don't understand the bigger picture and how things work, it will set us up for failure over the long run. Because just being told what to do stops working the minute we're bored of the workout plan, the meal plan, or information you've been handed. I, myself, didn't break through my 30-year struggle until I understood how the body and metabolism work at a deeper level.

So, to my fellow cut-to-the-chasers, no worries. You will learn the exact nuts and bolts of how to sweat, eat, and sleep very shortly. But to properly set the stage for the workouts, meals, and recovery you will do, I'm going to teach you some indispensable lessons about how metabolism works and common mistakes to avoid that can inadvertently slow your metabolism. Then, we'll go over the right way to elevate your metabolism. A lot of this is stuff you've either probably never learned before or never knew how to put together in a useful way.

Let's dive in!

THE POWERFUL BENEFITS OF A HAVING A FASTER METABOLISM

Transforming your body and maintaining it where you want it boils down to one essential skill: ***learning how to elevate your metabolism and keeping it high over time.***

Elevating your metabolism—the right way—unlocks numerous life-changing benefits including: a leaner body, more energy, better health, and enhanced longevity.

Better yet, for an over-40 professional, it provides you with what I call:"wiggle room to not have to be perfect all the time." This means that:

- Client dinners or pizza with the kids won't affect your waistline.
- On date night, you get to order anything on the menu worry-free.
- Business trips or days full of back-to-backs won't set you back.
- Weddings, holidays, and birthdays won't hurt your progress.
- You'll get to enjoy your favorite food and drink without guilt or remorse.

Sounds almost too good to be true, right? Well, it is true. These benefits are part of my reality, and I enjoy living with these freedoms on a daily basis. More importantly, my clients also get to enjoy these benefits and freedoms too. By using the *Nine Shifts* framework to consistently maintain their metabolism-boosting habits, it has provided them with (in their actual words):

- "confidence, energy, stamina, and vigor"
- "resilience, optimism, and purpose"
- "relief, clarity, calm, and control"
- "health, mobility, longevity, and independence"
- "peace of mind, enthusiasm, and the pride of accomplishment"

In essence, you'll look, feel, and perform your best.

Developing this skill will also future-proof you because, as you know by now, our metabolism slows as we age, especially after we hit our forties.

But elevating your metabolism, and keeping it high, is easier said than done. To give you the best chance of elevating your metabolism and enjoying these benefits, it's important to have at least a basic understanding of how the metabolism works.

A HIGH-LEVEL OVERVIEW OF METABOLISM

Just like with the mind, the metabolism has one primary mission: to ensure your survival.

The main way it does this is by making sure you never run out of energy.

Simply put, energy is required for life. If we go without energy for too long, we die. To make sure we never run out of energy, the metabolism is constantly monitoring: a) how much energy is coming in versus b) how much energy is going out.

Maintaining equilibrium between the two sides of this equation is a process known as energy balance. The metabolism will regulate and adjust how much energy it's making available based on how much energy we're giving it (via the food we're eating) versus how much we're using. When we provide the body with ample energy, it will make more energy available for use. When we don't, it will pull back on how much energy it makes available for our body to use, and will deprioritize energy for certain functions in favor of activities needed for safety and survival.

Most people are aware that if we eat more than we burn, the body will store the additional energy as fat. Conversely, if we burn more than we eat, the body makes up for the shortfall in energy by drawing on fat stores. (This is partly true, but not entirely true. More on this soon).

The energy coming in, measured in calories (kcal), comes from three different sources: protein, fats, and carbohydrates.

The energy going out, called Total Daily Energy Expenditure (TDEE), is spread across four categories.[41] We expend energy for everything from breathing, moving, thinking, digesting food, exercising, and beyond. The table and corresponding chart show the breakdown of calories by energy consumption source.

As you can see, the biggest contributor to how much energy one uses is the Basal Metabolic Rate (BMR). It accounts for about 60% (and as high as 80%) of the total calories we burn each day. One thing to note is that calories via our BMR are being burned while we're at rest (i.e., not during exercise

METABOLIC ENERGY CONSUMPTION

Energy Consumption Source	Approximate Share of Calories Burned	Purpose
Basal Metabolic Rate (BMR)	60%	Energy used for bodily functions and systems like breathing, thinking, heart beating, cell regeneration, etc.
Exercise Activity Thermogenesis (EAT)	10%	Energy used during formal exercise.
Non-exercise Activity Thermogenesis (NEAT)	20%	The energy expended for everything we do that is not sleeping, eating, or sports-like exercise.
Thermic Effect of Food (TEF)	10%	The amount of energy it takes for your body to digest, absorb, and metabolize the food you eat.

Note: These percentages are approximations and can vary by individual due to age, sex, genetics, activity level and other variables.

or physical activity). Our BMR is primarily given by our age, height, sex, and body fat percentage.[42] Because it's given by factors outside of our control such as genetics and age, BMR is harder to affect directly. Conversely, calories burned from

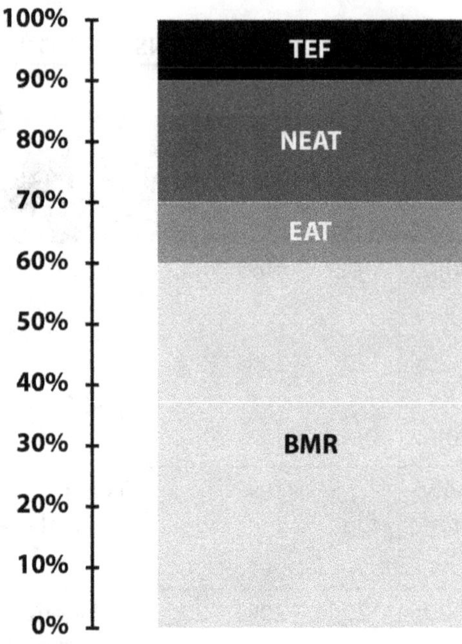

exercise are directly in our control because we get to say how long and how hard we'll go. But keep BMR in mind because elevating this number gives you the biggest bang for your buck when it comes to boosting your metabolism. Shortly, I will reveal the right way to speed up this important number so you can burn more calories, even at rest.

For now, let's review two features of the metabolism that are pertinent to our body transformation goals.

THE METABOLISM IS NOT STATIC

When it comes to the goal of transforming one's body, the thing that many people fail to realize is that our metabolism is not static. It does not burn the exact same number of calories every single day. It's constantly adjusting the number of calories being burned in response to a number of variables. This is one reason why basing one's weight loss or body transformation goal on a specific calorie consumption number (e.g., "just eat 1,200 calories and you'll lose weight") will not always work. Always eating a fixed number of calories when the metabolism could be burning more or less than that number creates a mismatch.

To understand what else we need to consider besides the calories we're consuming, let's look at the other factors, or inputs, that impact our metabolism.

THE METABOLISM LOOKS AT MORE THAN JUST CALORIES WE CONSUME

The metabolism considers many different inputs when deciding how much energy to make available for use (i.e., the calories it burns). Now, the amount of food coming in (calories we consume) is certainly one of the key inputs it looks at. After all, its job is to manage energy. Calories coming in makes up one side of the energy balance equation.

Energy Balance = Calories Coming In vs. Calories Going Out

But, unlike what you may have heard, energy coming in is not the only input the metabolism considers. In other words, when it comes to impacting our metabolism, calories are ***not*** all that matter.

In reality, the metabolism is constantly adjusting energy usage based on numerous inputs that consider what's going on around us (stress) as well as what's happening inside of us (our hormonal levels).

One of my mentors, Sam Miller, founder of the Metabolism School and author of the book *Metabolism Made Simple*[43] puts it this way: "(The metabolism) is constantly scanning and observing our external environment for stressors, while simultaneously evaluating our internal hormone levels using a system of checks and balances."

Inputs that impact our metabolism include, but are not limited to: stress of any kind (emotional, physical, environmental), quality of sleep and recovery, quality of nutrition, inflammation levels, hydration, digestion (including digestive issues), hormonal balances, and insulin sensitivity (or insulin resistance).[44] [45] [46] [47] [48] All of these variables play a role in the usage or storage of energy. So, when any of these inputs are outside of an optimal range, the metabolism will create adaptations in the body to account for them. A common example is when stress is high.

As we learned in Chapter 10, "Challenge #7: High Stress," chronically elevated stress levels increase cortisol and put us into "fight or flight" mode. In response to the stress it perceives, the metabolism will reduce the amount of energy it normally makes available for other functions (e.g., thinking, digestion, reproduction) to allocate more energy to help you fight off an attacker or run away. Thus, it will reduce how many calories it's burning overall in order to allocate energy towards helping you deal with the fight or flight situation. This is an example of the metabolism adjusting the rate at which it burns calories independently of the number of calories you ate that day.

In sum, our metabolism is reliant on numerous inputs and is constantly adapting to them. Thus, the number of calories we burn is constantly changing. To successfully impact our metabolism, we have to think beyond just a fixed calorie number and consider the numerous other factors that impact the metabolism, such as the demands being placed on it by things such as stress, poor sleep, inadequate nutrition, being sedentary, and the like. Because most people are not aware of this, they do not account for it and they fail in their attempt to elevate their metabolism and create lasting change.

They also make other mistakes that hurt their efforts to elevate their metabolism and transform their body.

COMMON MISTAKES PEOPLE MAKE WHEN TRYING TO ELEVATE THEIR METABOLISM

Let's look at some other common mistakes people make when trying to elevate their metabolism. Most people fall prey to the following missteps:

1. CUTTING CALORIES (DIETING)

While cutting calories can result in some initial weight loss it's not effective over the long run. As you know now, metabolism operates under the law of energy balance and will reduce the energy being burned if the energy coming in does not support the energy needs of the body. In other words, if we undereat for too long, the metabolism will slow down so it can burn less and preserve energy for your survival. This is why 90% of diets fail and any fat lost during the diet is usually regained, if not more.[49]

2. BURNING CALORIES (WITH CARDIO)

Cardio is popular for two reasons. First because it feels more familiar and less intimidating than, say, weight training. Second, because people have heard it burns more calories than other exercises or activities. Yes, doing cardio results in more calories burned during your session than other exercise modalities. It also helps you break a sweat which can feel good.

However, traditional, steady-state cardio does little to impact your resting metabolic rate once the session is over. Unless you're doing HIIT-style (High-Intensity Interval Training) cardio, which can be too intense for many people over-40, it can take significant amounts of traditional cardio like jogging to see changes in body fat levels.

3. EATING HEALTHIER

While eating healthier is always a good thing, in principle, people can often get it wrong. Having foods that seem healthy can drive up calories more than we realize. Yes, things like avocados, olive oil, and nuts are nutritious, but have too much and they'll quickly drive up your fat and caloric intake. Sure, smoothies have many vitamins and minerals. They're also full of sugar and can spike your insulin, leading to extra body fat.

This is not to say these foods are bad, merely that they have to be incorporated strategically. Otherwise, they can lead to a common gripe: "I don't understand why I'm not losing any weight! I eat so healthy!"

4. SHORTCUTS

This is a catch-all category to cover any get-thin-quick gimmicks like overhyped supplements, fancy fat loss injections, and BS biohacks. Going into the pros and cons of these approaches is beyond the scope of this book. Let me greatly simplify things for you by saying that most of these things don't live up to the hype the product makers want you to believe. Most have minimal impact on the metabolism, and those that do, like fat loss injection, have side-effects and result in regaining the weight once you stop using them.

Ultimately, there is no "shortcut" to a faster metabolism. You have to do the right things.

HOW TO KEEP YOUR METABOLISM ELEVATED THE RIGHT WAY

These three strategies are proven to elevate your metabolism in the most effective and lasting way.

1. **Adding muscle through strength training**—Muscle tissue is metabolically active. Having more of it elevates your resting metabolic rate and helps you burn more calories around the clock. We will tackle this in Chapter 19, "Shift #4: Train For Strength."
2. **Optimizing your nutrition for metabolism**—This is a combination of eating the right foods, at the right times, in the right quantities. With enough of the right nutrition coming in, you will support your training properly, optimize your hormones, and keep your metabolism high. We will tackle this in Chapter 20, "Shift #5: Optimize Your Nutrition."

3. **Sleeping and recovering properly**—Sleep is often overlooked but plays a huge role in metabolism and overall health. By using some simple tactics you will improve your sleep, keep your metabolism up, and your body fat down. We will tackle this in Chapter 21, "Shift #6: Enhance Your Sleep."

These are the three shifts you're about to make in the next three chapters.

By implementing the *Nine Shifts* Metabolism components you give yourself the best chance of having a faster metabolism and the benefits that come with it. Plus, by implementing the Mind and Momentum parts of the book, you'll ensure internal and external obstacles don't knock you off track so you can keep your metabolism elevated for years to come.

Happy faster metabolism for life.

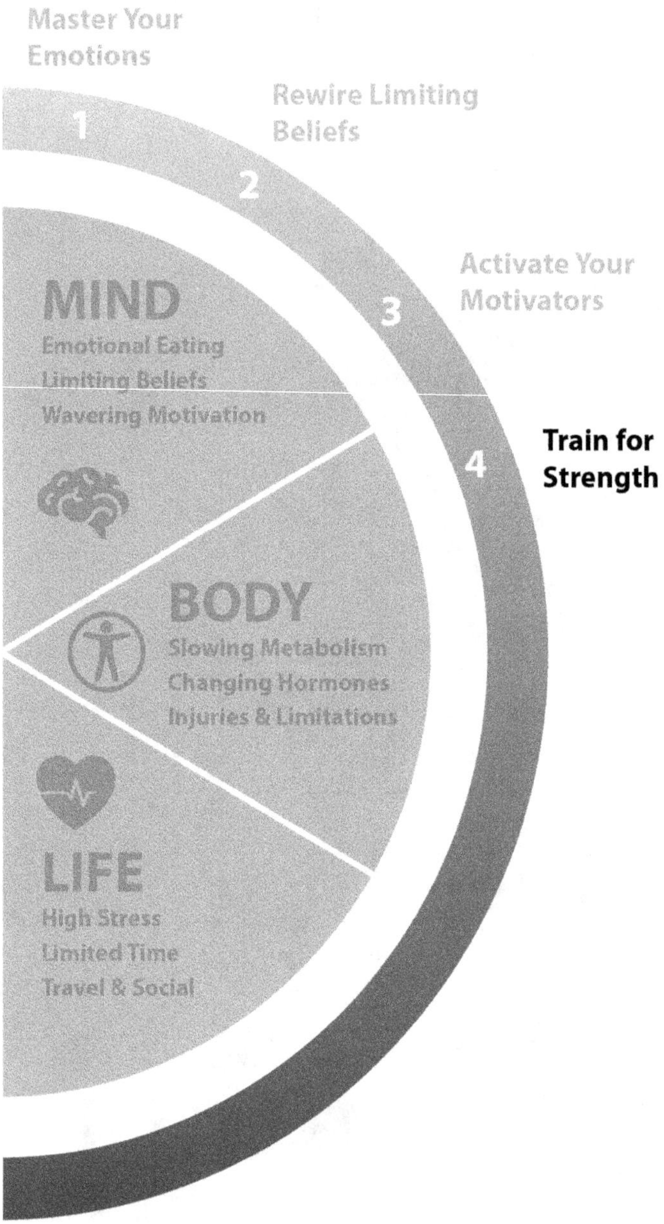

Master Your Emotions

Rewire Limiting Beliefs

Activate Your Motivators

Train for Strength

1
2
3
4

MIND
Emotional Eating
Limiting Beliefs
Wavering Motivation

BODY
Slowing Metabolism
Changing Hormones
Injuries & Limitations

LIFE
High Stress
Limited Time
Travel & Social

CHAPTER 19

SHIFT #4: Train for Strength

"The purpose of training is to tighten up the slack, toughen the body, and polish the spirit."
—Morihei Ueshiba

Metabolism elevation loading...

If our goal is to transform the body and become optimal by cutting fat, getting stronger and elevating our metabolism, then training for strength plays an essential role in delivering these outcomes in an effective and lasting way. Most people make mistakes in the area of their training, including making cardio their main form of exercise, undertraining, or not training consistently enough. In fact, according to the CDC only 31% of US adults met the recommended guidelines for muscle-strengthening activity.[50] In order get this step right, here is the key shift you will make:

KEY SHIFT

Go from doing lots of cardio or not training intensely or consistently enough, to training in a way that safely builds muscle and maintains muscle, in minimal time.

For our purposes, the biggest benefit of performing strength training is its ability to elevate our metabolism. It does this in multiple ways:

- First, by creating what's known as "metabolic stress" during our workout. This means strength training burns calories while we're exercising.
- Second, by triggering what's known as the "afterburn" effect. This keeps our metabolism elevated, and keeps us burning calories, for many hours after the strength training session is over. (More on this soon.)
- Third, by creating the stimulus we need to add more lean muscle tissue. Because muscle is metabolically active, the more of it we have, the higher our resting metabolic rate will be and the more calories we will burn throughout the day (even at rest).[51]

METABOLISM MATH: HOW TO BURN MORE CALORIES AROUND THE CLOCK

When we talk about body composition, we're referring to how much muscle and how much fat a person has. From a metabolic standpoint, having more muscle is what we want because muscle burns three times more energy than stored body fat does.

A pound of muscle burns approximately 6 calories per day at rest, while a pound of fat burns only 2 calories per day at rest.

This means by adding one additional pound of muscle you would burn 6 additional calories per day. What's more, moving a body that's heavier requires more energy. In other words, being one pound heavier (i.e., due to the additional pound of muscle you've gained) requires a higher active energy expenditure of 3–4 calories burned per extra pound of muscle you carry.[52]

ADDITIONAL CALORIES BURNED PER POUND OF MUSCLE

	1 lb of Muscle	10 lb of Muscle
Additional calories burned per day per additional pound of muscle tissue	6 calories	60 calories
Additional calories burned per day from higher active energy	3–4 calories	30–40 calories
Total additional calories burned per day	9–10 calories	90–100 calories

**Numbers above are approximations and can vary by person*

In sum, adding one additional pound of muscle results in 9–10 more calories burned per day. Now, if you were to add 10 lb of lean muscle over time, you'd become the proud owner of a metabolism that burns an extra 90–100 calories per day, before accounting for any exercise.

Not earth shattering, but not bad either.

Over the course of a week, that's an extra 600–700 extra calories burned. Enough to give you a cushion to easily enjoy things like a client dinner, a happy hour, or a date night without having them affect your waistline.

This is how having a faster resting metabolism gives you flexibility to not have to be perfect all the time.

If you've ever had to count every calorie, restrict your favorite foods, or couldn't help but feel guiltier than a Catholic nun during confession after a night out of eating and drinking with your friends, a faster metabolism will feel like a godsend.

Again, the key is adding some muscle to your frame.

Now, I'm not saying you need to turn into Arnold Schwarzenegger, unless you want to, of course. ("I'll be baaah-ck!") But I am saying to get your strength training and muscle-building dialed in so you can enjoy the wiggle room and flexibility that having a faster resting metabolism provides.

MUSCLE BRINGS MANY BENEFITS BEYOND CALORIE BURN

Besides elevating our metabolism and helping us stay lean, having more muscle also brings numerous powerful benefits including better mobility and performance, increased energy levels, more strength and stamina, as well as a more aesthetic appearance and the confidence that comes with it.

As you will soon see, both strength training and building muscle deliver tremendous health and life benefits. I trust that by reading about these benefits you will feel more incentivized and open to making strength training a regular part of your weekly routine, even if you haven't been an athlete or very active in your life. I believe that there is an athlete in everyone of us, and with the right approach, that athlete inside of you can emerge.

Our bodies were designed to move and to lift stuff.

On this note, I'll share what my client, Carla, the CEO of a Napa-based winery, said about getting back into strength training with our *Nine Shift* strength training approach:

"I have to say, one of the greatest things about this program is that it treats us like athletes, and not like 'overweight people,' which can be so stigmatizing and demotivating. I've been regaining a lot of confidence by doing the strength training, thinking about all of the good stuff I'm going to be able to do soon (like get back on the bike and play tennis again), and it's a mental win-win thought cycle."

THE APPROACH

To elevate our metabolism, the goal of our training will be to challenge the body to get stronger and build new muscle tissue.

The way to add lean muscle tissue is to train hard enough to tear down muscle fibers and then eat and recover properly so that your body replaces the muscle that was lost with new, thicker fibers that will withstand that same level of exertion better the next time you train.[53]

Tearing down muscle fibers may sound scary but it's actually a normal, natural adaptation the body undergoes to protect itself. It creates thicker fibers to handle the stress that's being placed on it, similar to how the body produces a blister (i.e., thicker skin) on your foot when there's too much friction from walking in shoes that are too tight.

The body's adaptive response to muscles being placed under challenging loads is to add thicker muscle fibers. This makes us stronger and elevates our metabolism. But it has to be done properly, and it has to be supported with proper nutrition and recovery.

Building muscle takes more than just throwing some dumbbells around.

Trust me, I tried that for 30 years and it didn't work, so let me spare you the frustration and the injuries.

As an aside, if this process sounds intimidating, hang in there. It's not as daunting or difficult as it may seem. The rest of this chapter and the Strength Training Plan coming up will make the process of adding muscle feel more friendly and attainable.

The Strength Training Plan was designed to be efficient, effective, adaptable, and safe on your joints. Its goal is to build strength, elevate the metabolism, and bulletproof the (aging) body in minimal time per week.

All it takes is three proper strength training workouts per week, for about 30–45 minutes, to keep our metabolism elevated, our muscles strong, and our body, and mind, running well.

For my cardio lovers, I'm not here to rain on your parade but, for our purposes of transforming the body in an optimal way, we have to prioritize strength training over cardio. That being said, I realize that cardio does have its benefits and can be enjoyable. I've always relished a good outdoor run or bike ride myself. To this end, the plan will show you how to incorporate cardio into the overall exercise approach.

The training principles below are considered to be the gospel of building muscle. Abide by these key principles if you want to add lean muscle and boost your metabolism in minimal time per week.

USE COMPOUND MOVEMENTS

A compound movement is an exercise that engages more than one muscle group at a time. A well-known example is a push-up, which engages your chest, triceps, and shoulders to help push you away from the floor. Other examples of popular compound movements include a squat, a lunge, a pullup, and a row.

By training multiple muscle groups simultaneously, employing compound movements cuts down on the time we need to spend on our workouts. Not only do compound movements allow you to finish your workout sooner, but also are more intense and place greater overall stress on the metabolism, elevating it to meet the higher intensity demands these movements place on our body.

The metabolic and hormonal adaptations that occur as a result of compound movements are far superior to that of isolation exercises (e.g., a bicep curl).

To maximize your results and save time, use compound movements for 80–100% of your training.

The Strength Training Plan features compound movements that will take you through a complete, full body workout that trains all major muscle groups in around 30–45 minutes, start to finish.

TRAIN TO FAILURE

A reporter once asked boxing legend Muhammad Ali how many sit-ups he performed per day. Ali gave an epic response: "I only start counting when it starts hurting because they're the only ones that count." This is the gist of what it means to train to failure. When it starts to burn is when it starts to work.

In essence, when we train to momentary muscle failure, we are safely pushing our muscles to the point of being fully fatigued and we can not perform another proper repetition with strict form.

To see how this works, let's bring back the pushup example. One repetition, or "rep" of the pushup is considered one full movement where you lower yourself down to the floor and then push away from the floor back up to the starting position. Once you do a certain number of reps of an exercise, that's considered one "set".

Let's say you begin doing push-ups and you easily complete the first five reps.

By the 6th rep, it starts to feel harder.

By the 7th rep, it's even harder, and you start feeling the burn.

By the 8th rep, your mind's comfort zone kicks in and says, "no more, please."

Except your body still has some effort left to give, and if you were to dig deep, you can probably squeeze out one or two more reps.

If you do, and you take this set of pushups to nine or even ten repetitions—to the point where your muscles truly become too weak to do another rep—then you've achieved momentary muscle failure. (Congratulations! You've activated progress!)

Training like this, combined with the right nutrition and recovery, helps us build more muscle and elevate our resting metabolic rate so we can burn more calories around the clock, even at rest.

Another thing that training in this fashion does is it challenges you, both physically and mentally, enabling you to become stronger in both body and mind.

Want to know what else training to failure does? (This is big . . .)

TRIGGERING THE AFTER BURN EFFECT

Training to failure triggers what's called EPOC—Excess Post-Exercise Oxygen Consumption. This is an "afterburn" effect that elevates your metabolism and keeps burning calories long after our workout is over. By applying this type of intensity during our strength training sessions[54] we create metabolic stress and elevate our metabolism, keeping it high for anywhere from 3–24 hours after the workout is over.[55]

Triggering EPOC is one of the most impactful and proven ways to elevate your metabolic burn. According to sports orthopedist James Larson III, MD, "Working at high intensity to failure is the best way to supercharge your metabolism."[56]

Now, you don't have to take every one of your sets to this level of intensity. There are actually different schools of thought on how many sets one should take to failure or how often. From my experience, if you can hit failure or get close to it on the majority of your working sets (i.e., your non-warmup sets), you will see significant improvement in body composition, strength, and mental fortitude in a short period of time.

Conversely, stopping well short of failure can result in limited progress.[57]

This being said, I realize that it's not always enjoyable to push ourselves (your mind's comfort zone will resist it), but the payoff for your effort is a stronger, leaner, and more vibrant you, in minimal time per week. It requires a focused mindset and a willingness to push beyond the point of where things start to get uncomfortable. Like author Fred Devito says, "If it doesn't challenge you, it doesn't change you."

Personally, I like to push myself to safely achieve momentary muscle failure, or at least get very close, on the majority of my working sets. Consistently challenging myself this way during exercise has paid big dividends in strengthening my body and my mind, priming me to take on other challenges that business and life have thrown my way.

PRACTICE PROGRESSIVE OVERLOAD

There's a fable about a Greek boy named Milo of Croton who lived in the 6th century B.C. Milo wanted to be an Olympic wrestler when he grew up. Knowing that he had to get stronger, he started carrying around a calf that had been recently born near his home. Every day, Milo would hoist the calf and carry it around. As time went on, the animal grew bigger and heavier. As a result, Milo became stronger and stronger because he was carrying around an animal that progressively got heavier and heavier. This strategy worked so well that Milo went on to become a six-time wrestling champion at the Olympic games in Greece!

Now, you may or may not be looking to become an Olympic wrestler, but the moral of the story is that if you want to progress over time, you must steadily increase the loads with which you're working. This is the principle of progressive overload.

You can do this by either adding more weight to your exercises or keeping the weight the same but doing more repetitions per set.

For simplicity, let's say you complete ten repetitions on the leg press machine at a resistance of 100 lb. This amount of weight feels challenging but doable, and it takes you pretty close to failure.

The following week (let's call it "Week #2), you will set the machine at a slightly heavier weight, say 110 lb, and try to perform the same ten repetitions with this higher weight.

Alternatively, you can keep the weight at 100 lb of resistance on the machine, the same as it was last week, but try to perform more repetitions this time, doing eleven or twelve reps with the same 100 lb of resistance instead of the ten you did last week.

During your Week #2 workout, whether you do the same ten repetitions with 110 lb of weight or keep the weight at 100 lb but perform more than ten repetitions, you've gotten stronger in both cases. This creates more strength, metabolic stress, muscle damage, and, in turn, even more elevation of your metabolism.

Every one to two weeks, you will try to do a little more in terms of repetitions or the weight you're using to ensure you keep getting stronger and continue adding more metabolism-boosting muscle.[58]

THE STRENGTH TRAINING PLAN

GUIDELINES:

- Time Required: 30–45 minutes
- What You Will Need: Depending on your level, all you will need is a pair of resistance bands with handles or an adjustable dumbbell set.
- There are workouts for three levels of exercise. Choose your starting program:
    - **Beginner**—For those coming back from a long lay off or not very experienced with weight training.
    - **Intermediate**—For those who have been exercising regularly and would like to focus more on strength training.

INTERMEDIATE & ADVANCED TRAINING PLANS

The beginner routine is on the pages that follow. The intermediate and advanced workout routines, along with other resources, are at this link: https://thenineshifts.com/downloads

- **Advanced**—Have been doing some kind of resistance training—body weight, machines, free weights—regularly.

- Start with the level at which you feel most comfortable. Perform the routine three days per week until you feel ready to progress to the next level.
- The workouts can be performed at home, at a gym, or in a hotel room.
- If you enjoy cardio exercises, by all means, feel free to add jogging, cardio machines, or fitness classes to this routine, once or twice per week, in addition to—not instead of—your strength workouts; strength training is foundational.

- Each workout starts with a functional warm up and joint mobilization designed to prepare you for the strength movements in the workout routine.
- You will finish each workout with core work, a quick cardio session, and a light stretch at the end.

Notes:

- Muscle soreness after a workout is normal. Muscles will be less sore after your workouts over time.
- If you feel stiffness and tightness in your joints such as shoulders, hips, or lower back, go slow and listen to your body. Training through a little pain or stiffness may be OK, but if the pain becomes chronic, it is best to get it checked by a physical therapist or healthcare professional.
- Train safely with good form but do push yourself a bit more with every workout.
- Remember that by using this plan, and any information in this book, you agree to do so at your own risk.

Pro Tip: I recommend you track your workout data (exercises, sets, and reps) on a small notebook or on a note in your phone. This makes it easy to remember where you left off the last time in terms of the pounds/kilos you used. It also allows you to see how you're progressing and getting stronger over time, which will motivate you to do more!

WARM UP

1 **Arm Hug**	10 hugs; alternate top arm each time	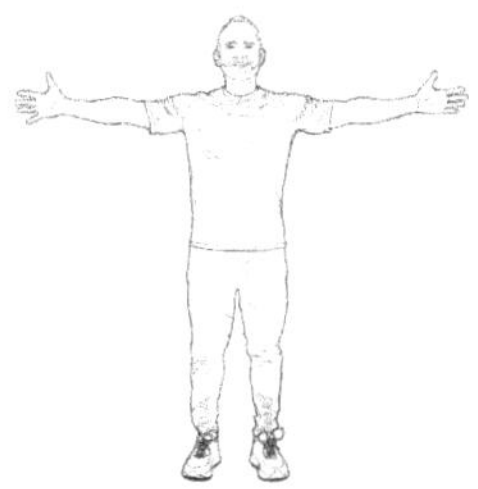
2 **Arm Circle**	5-10 seconds each direction	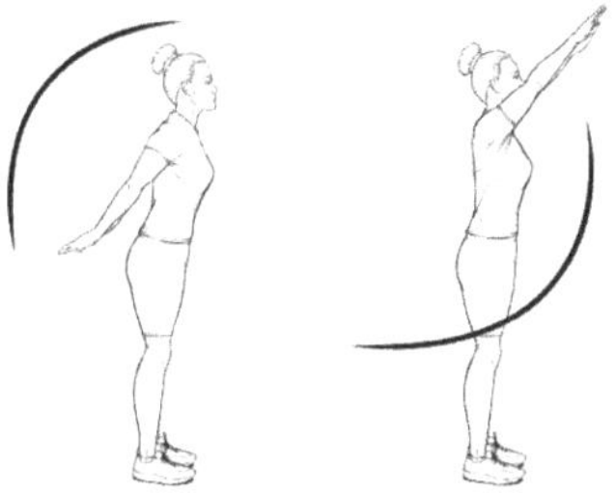
3 **Dynamic Wall Dog**	2 sets x 6-8 repetitions	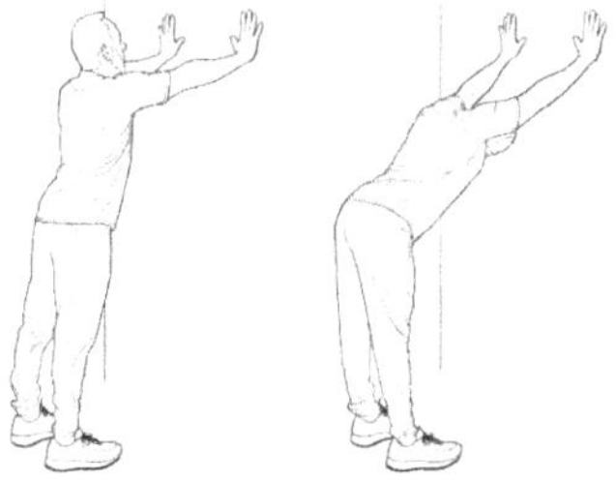
4 **Dynamic Hip Flexor Stretch**	5-10 second hold per side	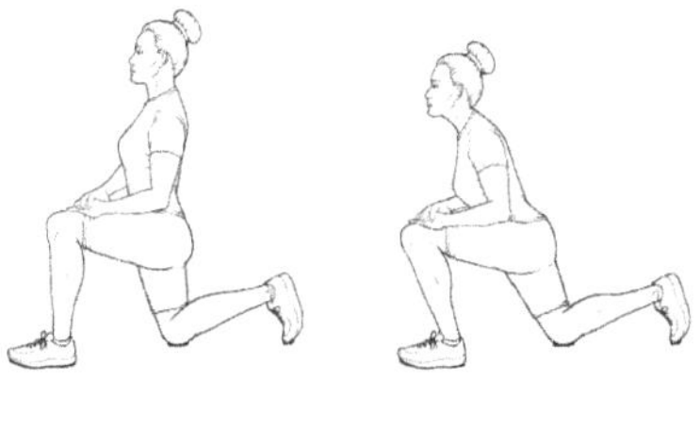

5 **Hip Hinge to Wall**	2 sets x 5-10; slow, gentle, brace your core through-out; rest 10 sec between sets	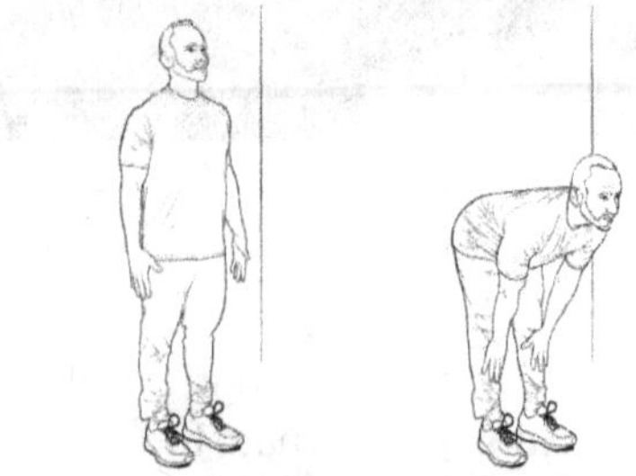

WORKOUT

1 **Half-Squat to Chair**	2 sets x 10-20 Rest 20 sec between sets	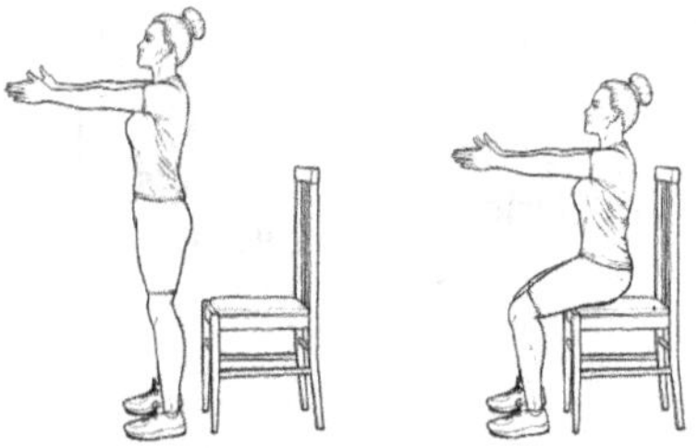
2 **Wall Sit**	3 sets x 10-15 seconds; rest 15 sec between sets	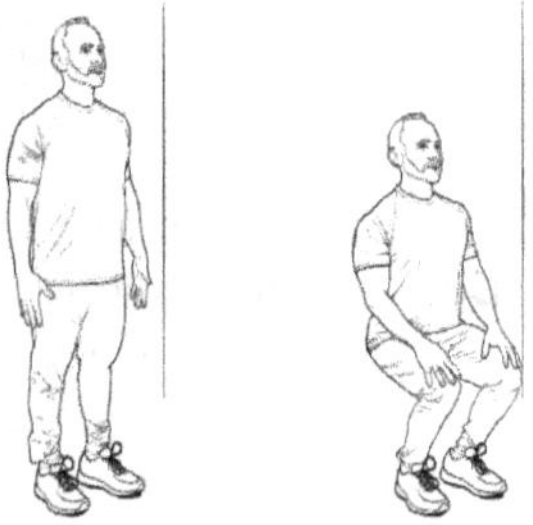
3 **Band Standing Row**	2 sets x 20-30; rest 30 sec between sets	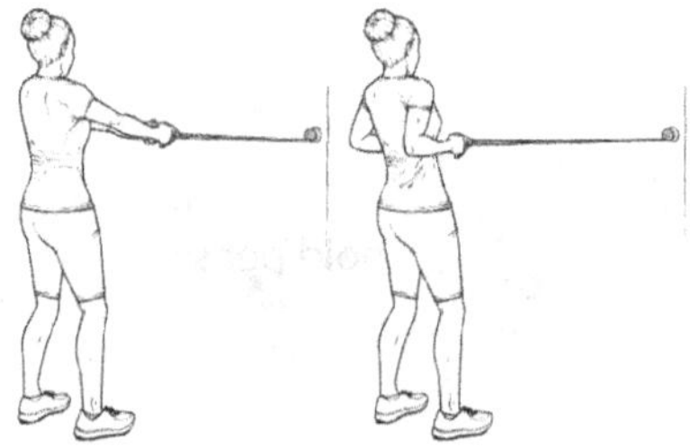

4 **Band Chest Press**	2 sets x 15-20; rest 30 sec between sets	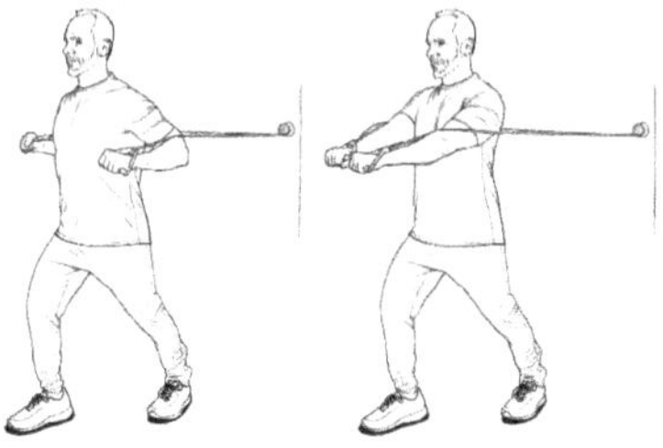
5 **Band Shoulder Press**	2 sets x 10-12; rest 30 sec between sets	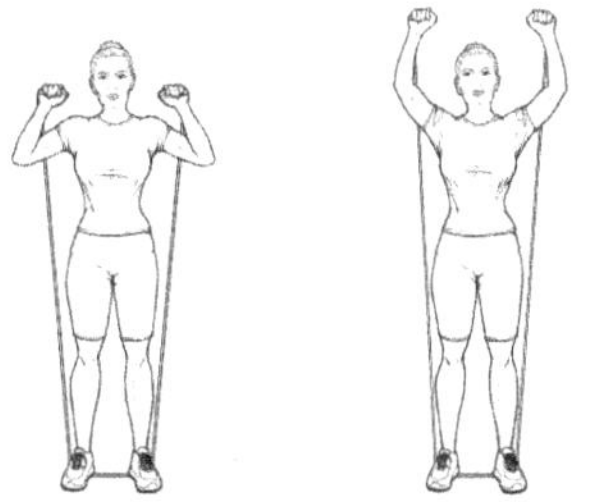
6 **Band Low-High Wood Chopper**	2 sets x 10-12 per side; rest 30 sec between sets	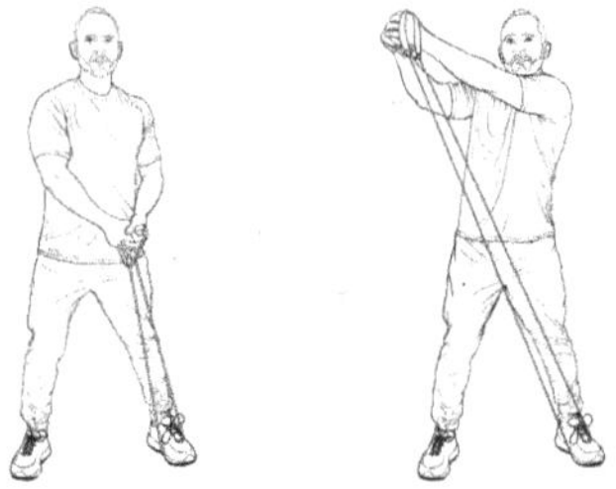

CORE WORKOUT

1 **Straight Leg Crunch**	2 sets x 10-15; rest 20 sec between sets	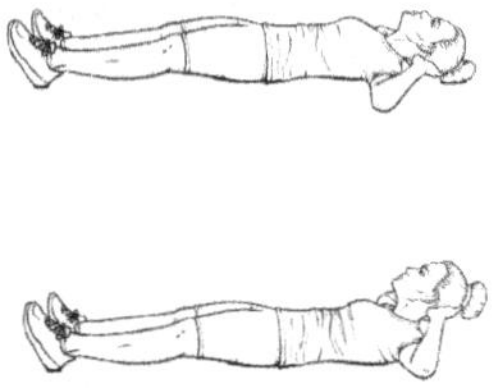
2 **Glute Bridge**	2 sets x 10-15; rest 20 sec between sets	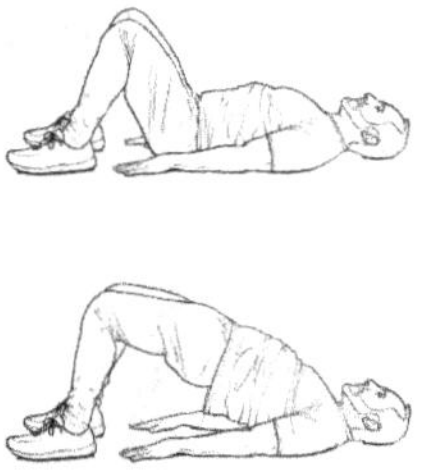

CARDIO FINISHER

Fast Feet	Run in place; pump your feet as quickly as you can 3 sets x 10 seconds on, 10 off	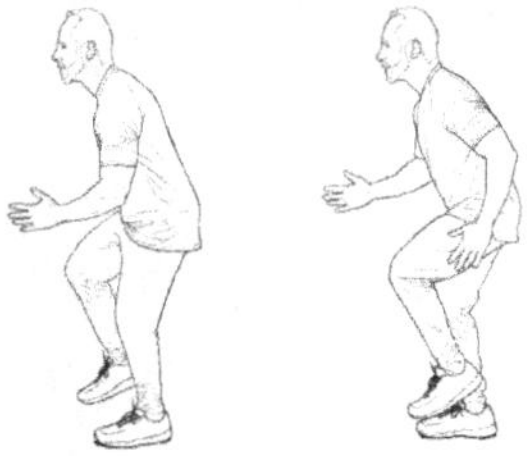

STRETCHING

1 **Seated Piriformis Stretch**	10-20 sec per side	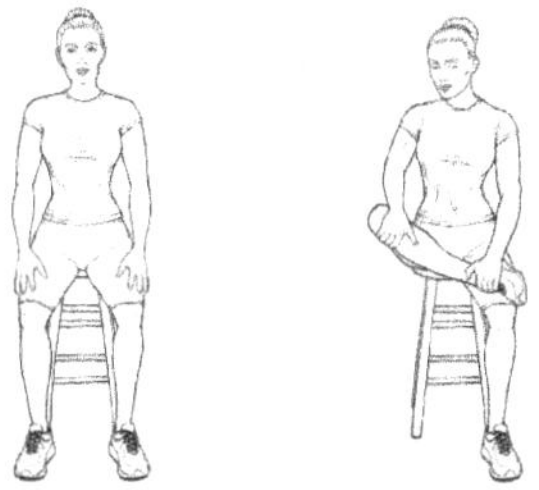
2 **Chest Opener**	5 second hold	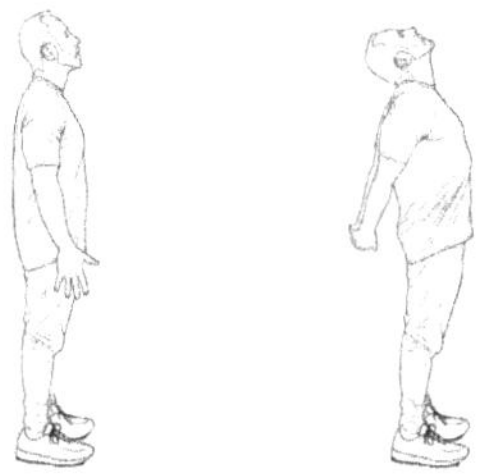
3 **Back Opener**	5 second hold per side	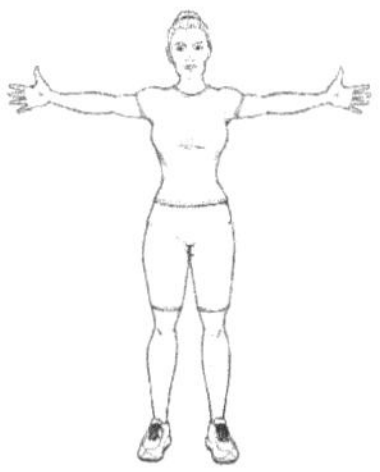

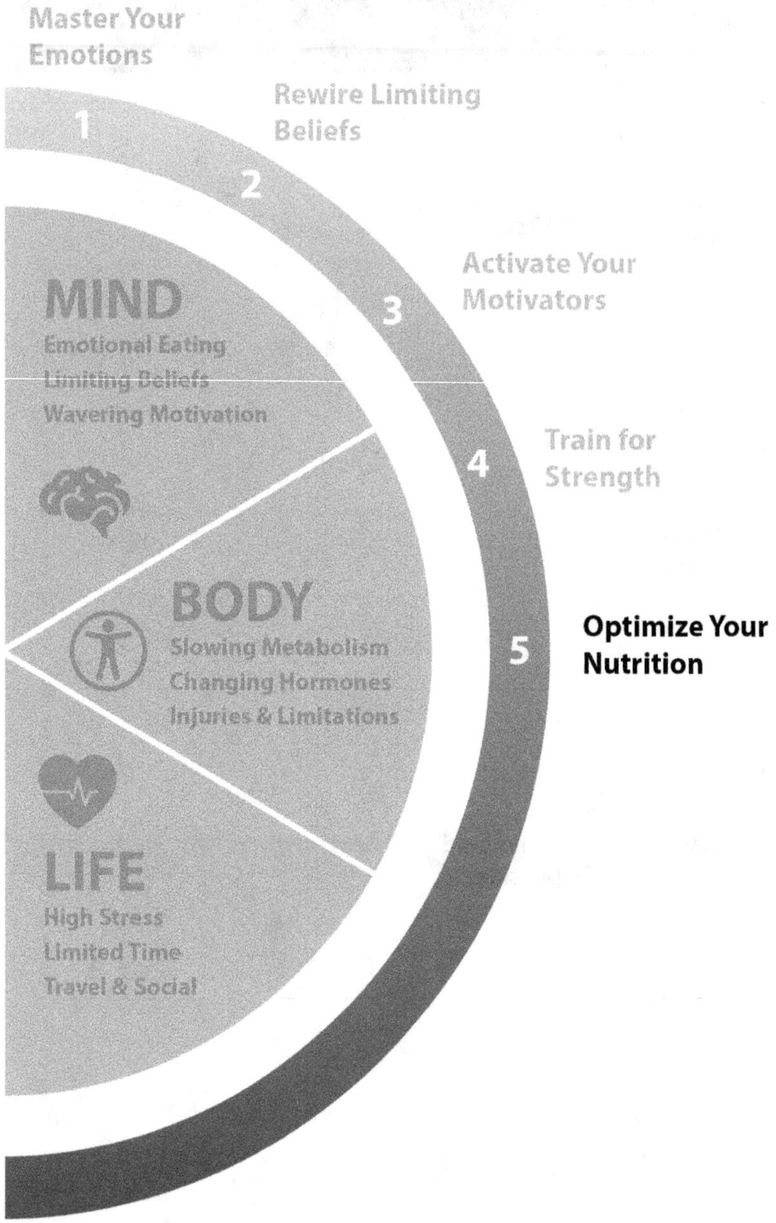

Master Your Emotions

1

Rewire Limiting Beliefs

2

Activate Your Motivators

3

MIND

Emotional Eating

Limiting Beliefs

Wavering Motivation

Train for Strength

4

BODY

Slowing Metabolism

Changing Hormones

Injuries & Limitations

5

Optimize Your Nutrition

LIFE

High Stress

Limited Time

Travel & Social

CHAPTER 20

SHIFT #5: Optimize Your Nutrition

"Our food should be our medicine, and
our medicine should be our food."
—Hippocrates

Now let's turn our attention to what might be, arguably, the single most important factor for elevating your metabolism and achieving a healthy, energized, and high-performing body: your nutrition.

Most people make mistakes in the area of their nutrition by doing things like dieting, eating strictly for pleasure, eating for convenience, or eating unconsciously. In order to get this step right, here is the key shift you will make:

KEY SHIFT

Go from cutting calories, undereating, and eating in an ad hoc manner to taking a more structured approach to your eating by having the right meals on hand to consume the right nutrition at the right times, with room for fun.

While nutrition is an essential part of the journey to a better body, it's also the area that the majority of people find the most challenging. Recent data suggest that 90% of Americans have a poor diet.[59]

Optimizing nutrition is the area that the majority of over-40 professionals struggle with the most.

I will confess that I, myself, didn't achieve impressive results in my body until I learned a good deal about nutrition and started keeping the right nutrition habits consistently.

There are numerous reasons getting our nutrition right can be challenging. First, there is much to learn when it comes to this topic because it's based in science and we don't learn much about it growing up. Second, there is an avalanche of information coming at us daily about what and how to eat, much of it conflicting. "Do Keto! No, eat plant based! No, eat Paleo! No, eat Carnivore! Have dairy! No, don't have dairy!", ad infinitum.

In other cases, nutritional information can be based on biased research or deceiving with hyped up claims in order to sell products. For instance, products claiming to be "packed with protein!" when, in reality, they merely have a nominal amount of low quality, low-bioavailable protein added for marketing purposes.

Other obstacles to getting our nutrition right include having to plan our meals, juggle eating with work and life, fight off cravings, and avoid the unhealthy foods that surround us.

THE APPROACH

The main objective of your nutritional approach will be to consume foods that will keep you healthy, while supporting the energy needs of your life.

Your food intake should also keep your metabolism high by fueling the kind of training that builds lean muscle and triggers the calorie-torching EPOC after burn effect. Your nutrition also has to help you recover properly from your workouts. In turn, you will have more muscle, be stronger, and have a faster metabolism.

It's important we get this shift right because:

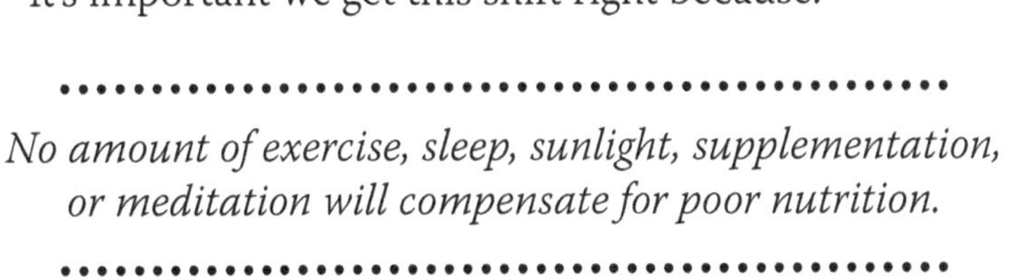

No amount of exercise, sleep, sunlight, supplementation, or meditation will compensate for poor nutrition.

That's why the fitness industry has a saying: "You can't outtrain a bad diet."

While getting this area right can be challenging, a simple way to optimize your nutrition is to eat the right foods, at the right times, in the right amounts. This means we have to manage all three aspects of our nutrition:

- what to eat (the right foods)
- when to eat (the right times)
- how much to eat (the right amounts)

Most people only focus on one of these aspects. They might focus on eating less ("how much to eat") or focus on eating only when they're hungry ("when to eat"). This one-sided approach is a big source of their body transformation struggles.

Starting now, you're going to take a different approach that will optimize all three aspects of nutrition and do it in a way that fits your schedule and palate, with enough leeway to have treat meals, some wine, or eating out with clients or friends.

TO OPTIMIZE YOUR NUTRITION, FOCUS ON:

WHAT YOU'RE EATING
WHEN YOU'RE EATING
HOW MUCH YOU'RE EATING

First, you will take back control of what you're eating by prepping your own meals. This will help you avoid having to always rely on outside food. This will give you more control and reduce the amount of processed foods you eat, keeping inflammation low and your hormones happy. By having the right foods already cooked and at the ready, you will be able to eat proper meals more quickly, so you can get it in and get back to business, even if you are on the road or juggling meetings all day.

Second, you will learn how to properly combine fats, carbs, and proteins and have them when it's most optimal. This will help sustain your energy levels and avoid the dreaded food coma, to keep your energy up and decision making sharp. It will also give your body opportunities to tap into stored body fat for energy instead of keeping blood sugar elevated all day long.

Third, you will no longer be overly restrictive in your approach to how much to eat. You will eat more than before and be properly nourished; never hungry or famished. Your nutrition will power you through your busy day and support your training and muscle-building efforts. This will give you a faster metabolism and plenty of flexibility to deal with one-off events or occasional treat meals where you eat and drink more than usual.

This will help change your relationship with food from one that is based on restriction and feeling remorse for non-adherence, to eating in control 80% of the time with room for guilt-free fun 20% of the time. This will result in balance and sustainability.

DESIGN OF THE NUTRITION OPTIMIZATION PLAN

The Nine Shifts Nutrition Optimization Plan is a simple, science-based strategy designed to help you keep your metabolism elevated, burn fat around the clock, get your body lean, and prime your health, without having to diet, eliminate your favorite foods, or put a lot of thought into what to eat for best results.

Best of all, it's flexible and sustainable. It's fluid enough to meet the needs of a busy professional, even if you are in meetings all day or traveling.

The Nutrition Optimization Plan is more than just a rigid meal plan, a strict diet, or a specific recipe. (I mean, who wants to eat grapefruit and cottage cheese every day? No thanks!)

Instead, it's an overall, flexible eating strategy that gives you freedom to have a wide range of foods. It also helps you make better choices when you are eating out or traveling, by guiding you on how to eat versus limiting you to specific foods only.

Earlier you met my client, Tammy, a 58-year old finance executive, and heard how she worked with us to transform her body, post-menopause. She lost a significant amount of excess body fat and shifted into feeling lighter and more energetic.

She credits the flexibility we gave her in how she could structure her meals as one of the main keys to her success. She says, "This wasn't restrictive, but it let me eat what I wanted as long as I stayed within my goals. I felt like I could adapt my eating while I traveled. I could just eat anything as long as I met my protein, fat, and carb goals that you laid out, and I liked that. I liked that A LOT."

THREE KEY NUTRITION PRINCIPLES

To get your nutrition optimized, be sure you're following these key nutrition principles. They're science-based and proven. They will help you take back control of your food, your body and your health. If you want to want be lean, healthy and energized, do this:

1. **What to eat:** stick to whole foods.
2. **When to eat:** limit insulin spikes.
3. **How much to eat:** hit your macros and micros.

Principle #1: Keep Inflammation Low by Sticking to Whole Foods

For a simple answer to the question "What should I eat?" you can follow this basic rule: eat whole foods.

To simplify your nutrition, stick to whole, unprocessed foods at least 80% of the time.

This means following these guidelines:

- Eating things like whole cuts of lean poultry, fish, meat, eggs, vegetables, fruits, and minimally processed, gluten-free grains like rice, quinoa, or oats.
- Having things like dairy in moderation.
- Limiting things like processed meats, breads and pastas, sugary drinks and sodas, fried foods, and baked sweets.

Sticking to these foods help us eat in line with how our bodies were designed. Unquestionably, the more aligned our food consumption is with how our body naturally functions, the better we will look, feel, and perform.

If you can't pick it, kill it, or grow it, it's best to limit it.

On the other hand, when we eat foods that are highly processed, such as refined carbs, it can negatively impact our hormones, gut health, and brain health. Harmful potential outcomes include a slower metabolism, excess body fat, reduced energy, increased risk of disease (including heart disease), suppressed immunity, mood swings, sleep disruption, inflammation, indigestion, and diminished cognitive function, including memory lapses; the list goes on.

While our bodies can handle processed foods from time to time, they're obviously not the most optimal. Thus, it's best to limit them, especially if your goal is to transform your body rapidly or to keep yourself healthy and at peak performance.

Principle #2: Limit Blood Sugar Spikes

As mentioned, it's essential for us to properly manage blood sugar (blood glucose) levels throughout our lives. This applies whether we already have prediabetes, Type 2 diabetes, or not. Being mindful of our blood sugar levels (and the carbs we eat) allows us to stay lean, enjoy sustained energy, and keep ourselves functioning properly and free from disease.

To keep blood sugar levels in check, we must ensure that we are limiting both the intensity and frequency of blood sugar spikes. Here's why.

The body will use either blood sugar or stored body fat for energy. When blood sugar is elevated (known as the "fed state"), the body uses this sugar for energy. When blood sugar is low (known as the "fasted state"), the body switches to using stored body fat for energy.

THERE IS NO "PERFECT" NUTRITION STRATEGY

I can hear the naysayers grumbling about some of the information in this chapter. To address any concerns, please allow me to compassionately say the following.

When it comes to nutrition, there are many different schools of thought and more opinions on the subject than Heinz got pickles. To the best of my knowledge, there isn't one "perfect" way of eating that everyone should follow, despite what many social media know-it-alls or study-touting science blowhards would like you to believe.

Every individual's metabolic profile is as unique as their fingerprint. Different foods affect people differently. That's why I'm not here to espouse what I think is the perfect nutrition strategy, diet, or eating style. Rather, I'm sharing the science-based best practices I've learned in my research and have seen work well for my clients and I in transforming our bodies. It's an approach that gets us to our goal of being lean, healthy, strong, and energized, while being practical and leaving room to enjoy food. I encourage everyone to learn more about the subject. Then, experiment and see how different foods make you feel and how they affect your body composition. Above all, make your nutrition work for you—your individual philosophy, palette and preferences. (That's the only "perfect" there is.)

We have to give the body a chance to alternate between using carbs for energy and stored body fat for energy.

Our goal is to allow the body to do its happy dance between burning carbs and burning stored body fat. This keeps our energy stable and our body lean. To maintain this balance between burning sugar and stored fat, we have to be strategic with our carbohydrate intake. That's because the carbs we eat elevate blood sugar levels more than any other macronutrient.

Now, this does not mean that carbs are the enemy or that we have to totally banish carbs from our diet. Despite what Keto zealots or Keto supplement peddlers may claim, carbs absolutely have their place in a balanced diet. In fact, carbs are the body's and brain's preferred energy source. We function and perform much better when we're strategically having the right carbs.

What most people do, unknowingly, is mismanage their carbs and keep blood sugar elevated throughout the day, never giving the body a chance to tap into stored body fat for energy.

They constantly spike blood sugar throughout the day by eating along these lines: having a bagel in the morning, a sandwich for lunch, a chocolate bar or pastry or coffee with sugar in the afternoon, and pasta for dinner.

This way of constantly having carbs keeps blood sugar consistently elevated and makes losing stubborn body fat seemingly even more stubborn. Furthermore, because insulin is required to store the carbs we're consuming, this way

THE 7 DEADLY SINFUL FOODS

In general, you want to limit or avoid what I playfully call "The 7 Deadly Sinful Foods."[60]

THE 7 DEADLY SINFUL FOODS

1. Processed meats (hot dogs, sausages, deli meats)
2. Fried foods (french fries, chips, fried rice)
3. Refined sugar and artificial sweeteners (table sugar, Splenda, Aspartame)
4. Soybean based products (tofu, soy milk, cheap mayo, cheap salad dressings)
5. Gluten (bread, pasta, beer, baked goods)
6. Corn and corn additives (corn syrup, dextrose, maltodextrin)
7. Vegetable oils especially if hydrogenated (Canola, palm, grapeseed, soybean, cotton-seed)

While I can't get into why each of these foods are not ideal (my editor will kill me if I make this chapter longer!) just know that these foods can either be inflammatory or can negatively affect our hormones and gut health. They've been linked to obesity, cancers, and other negative health outcomes. Ironically, most of these foods are found in abundance. Check the ingredient labels carefully when you shop and you'll see!

When it comes to shopping for whole unprocessed foods, keep in mind that U.S. food manufacturing and farming practices have been shown to use low-quality animal feed, antibiotics, hormones, and pesticides, among other contaminants.

Here are some guidelines to help you make the healthiest choices.

- buy organic chicken and eggs
- buy grass fed beef
- buy wild caught fish
- buy organic vegetables and fruits

These options can be more expensive (sometimes not by much) but investing in higher quality foods will be optimal for your health and energy levels and will pay back dividends in the form of less inflammation, reduced chances of illness, better mood, enhanced longevity, and overall performance.

of eating keeps insulin persistently elevated, which can lead to the beginning of insulin resistance and eventually Type 2 diabetes and metabolic syndrome.

Thus, our objective is to manage both the intensity and frequency of blood sugar spikes, like so:

- To reduce the ***intensity*** of blood sugar spikes, we are prompted to eat foods that have a limited impact on blood sugar levels. This includes eating lean protein (like white fish), healthy fat (like olive oil), and fibrous carbs (like brown rice or beans). The Nutrition Optimization Plan includes low glycemic carbs that have a smaller impact on your blood sugar levels. It also combines foods that limit the intensity of insulin spikes, particularly by adding fiber to slow the absorption of carbs into the bloodstream.

- To reduce the ***frequency*** of blood sugar spikes, we will limit the number of times we eat food, primarily carbs, during the day. One of the main ways to do this is called Time Restricted Eating (TRE), commonly known as Intermittent Fasting. The Nutrition Optimization Plan has TRE as one of its principles and limits carbs to a specific time window instead of spreading out your carb intake throughout the day.

In this way, you can see how this key nutrition principle of timing our meals and our carbs addresses when to eat.

Principle #3: Hit Your Macros & Micros

This third key principle helps address how much to eat. Like with everything else—exercise, sleep, etc.—we want to take a Goldilocks approach to our food. We don't want to eat too little, nor too much; we want to eat just right.

The foods we eat either contain macronutrients, micronutrients, or both. The macronutrients are proteins, carbohydrates, and fats. These are the only nutrients that contain calories. The micronutrients are primarily vitamins and minerals. They are ingested in much smaller quantities, but don't let that fool you. They, too, play a key role in how our body functions.

Hitting Your Macronutrient Targets

We want to ensure that we're hitting our recommended macronutrient targets as often as possible. That's because each macronutrient plays a key role in the body.

- **Protein**—builds lean muscle, elevates metabolism, and keeps all of our cells functioning properly.
- **Carbohydrates**—fuel us; are the preferred energy source for our body and brain.
- **Healthy Fats**—play a key role in the function of our hormones and our cells, aid in absorption of nutrients, and keep inflammation low.

Our focus will be getting the right amount of protein, fats, and carbohydrates each day. Since each one of these macronutrients contain calories, hitting our daily macro targets ensures we also hit our calorie goal for the day.

The easiest way to find your calorie goal and answer the question "How much should I eat?" is to use an online calculator that will estimate your Total Daily Energy Expenditure (TDEE) using scientific formulas. One such site I like to use is https://tdeecalculator.net.

Once you have your total daily calorie target, allocate the calories based on the different macronutrient percentages.

TDEE (as calculated online)	Calorie Adjustment (assuming weight loss goal)	Final Calorie Target (how much to eat each day)
2,500	-500	2,000
1,800	-500	1,300

For example, if the goal is weight loss, I suggest starting with an initial target of protein at 40%, carbs at 30% and fats at 30%. So for a 2,000 calorie diet, your breakdown would look like the table below (which has examples for two different caloric targets).

Then, to figure out how to hit these targets, divide them by the number of meals and snacks you will have each day. For example, if you will have breakfast, lunch and dinner, along with one snack, you want to have around 40g of carbs on average per meal to hit your daily carb target of 150g, and so on.

Logging your food for a few days with a food tracking app will show you how close or how far you are from hitting your macronutrient targets each day. With a little practice and fine-tuning of your meals, you'll get the hang of hitting your targets (and remember, we're only looking for 80% of the time; the other 20% you can freestyle and eat pretty much whatever you want).

Hitting Your Micronutrient Targets

Now that you know how to hit your macronutrients (protein, carbs, and fats), make sure you're eating enough fruits and vegetables each day to get your micronutrients (vitamins

Protein Target (40% of calories)	Fat Target (30% of calories)	Carb Target (30% of calories)
800 (200g)	600 (67g)	600 (150g)
520 (130g)	390 (43g)	390 (98g)

WHY PROTEIN IS THE KING OF MACRONUTRIENTS

For our purposes, protein is our best friend. First, because it's required for building muscle tissue. As mentioned, having more muscle results in a faster resting metabolic rate and a well-functioning body.

Second, because eating protein actually elevates our metabolism via the Thermic Effect of Food. Digesting food requires calories and breaking down protein requires more calories than any other nutrient. The body uses up to 30% of the protein calories ingested to break down that protein. This means that if you eat 100 calories in protein, the net caloric impact after digestion is only 70 calories.

The catch is, most people undereat protein. But by adding protein to every meal, and supplementing with protein powder when needed, you will start benefiting from this all-important macronutrient.

and minerals); this will also help you get fiber and stay regular. When short on time, you can supplement with a quality multivitamin or greens powder.

Finally, I'd be remiss to not at least mention hydration in this section of how much to consume. One of our medical advisors, Dr. Hatem Zayed, MD, a leading specialist in functional medicine and anti-aging, recommends we drink half our weight in ounces of water per day. So if someone weighs

150 lb, for example, they would drink 75 oz, or roughly 9 cups (or 2 liters) of water each day. Add more if in high altitude, high humidity, or doing strenuous activities or exercise.

THE NUTRITION OPTIMIZATION PLAN

GUIDELINES:

- Time Required: 1.5–2.5 hours to prep meals in a batch cooking fashion
- What You Will Need:
    - Basic cooking tools, such as a few baking dishes, some utensils, and a couple of pots.
    - You can also use an indoor or outdoor grill. Feel free to add things like food processors, rice cookers, or an air fryer; get as fancy or as no-frills as you'd like.
    - Download a food logging app like MyFitnessPal, LoseIt, or Cronometer to help track your calorie and macronutrient intake (they're free; recommended but not required).
- There is a meal plan for an entire day's worth of eating laid out across 3 meals and one snack.
    - Plan A is for a 50-year old female of average height (5'4") weighing 170 lb.
    - Plan B is for a 50-year old male of average height (5'9") weighing 200 lb.
- You can adjust calories up or down based on your current bodyweight (keep macro percentages the same).

- Both plans assume a goal of losing body fat and are set at a safe level of 500 calories below the Total Daily Energy Expenditure, which is based on the assumption that the person will do some light to moderate exercise.
- For a closer estimation of your required daily calories use this website to calculate your caloric needs: https://tdeecalculator.net.

Notes:

- You will have a slightly delayed breakfast (unless you work out first thing in the morning, in which case you can have a protein shake or eat breakfast after your workout). After that, you will have lunch and dinner, with a snack in between.
- To help reduce the number of insulin spikes during the day, the meal plan places your starchy carb intake during a 4–6 hour window.
- This is a suggested meal plan, not a customized one to your specific metabolism, palette, or schedule. Feel free to make adjustments in foods, quantities, and timing to make it sustainable for you.
- This plan is intended for fat loss and should provide some initial fat loss results. Over time, your metabolism may slow and you may hit a plateau. This will require strategically adding more calories and doing what's known as a "Reverse Diet" to ensure you continue losing body fat. It is suggested you work with a professional to guide you through this process because it can be tricky.

MEAL PLANS

FULL DAY OF EATING EXAMPLE: MEAL PLAN A–170 LB FEMALE

9 am—Breakfast

Protein + Fat, NO Starchy Carbs

- ☐ Veggie omelet or scrambled: 1 egg, 3 egg whites, veggies, non-stick spray
- ☐ 70%+ dark chocolate (1 serving)

Alternative breakfast strategy for when busy or traveling:

- ☐ 1 serving of protein powder (whey or egg) with water or almond milk (use blender or shaker cup), add greens powder, have with mixed nuts
- ☐ 70%+ dark chocolate (1 serving)

12 pm—Lunch

Protein + Carbs, Limit Fat

- ☐ 6 ounces of lean protein (chicken breast, tuna, cod, turkey breast, shrimp, white fish, etc.)
- ☐ 1.5 serving of healthy carbs (sweet potato, brown rice, quinoa, lentils, any kind of beans)

- ☐ Mixed veggies or spinach salad with light dressing

4 pm—Snack

Protein + Carbs, Limit Fat

- ☐ 1 serving of lean protein snack (organic beef jerky, tuna, or protein powder)
- ☐ 1 serving of steel cut oatmeal or fruit (berries, apple, orange, etc.)—can replace carbs with mixed nuts on non-training days)

7 pm—Dinner

Protein + Fat, Limit Carbs

- ☐ 6 ounces of fattier protein (salmon, steak, lamb, pork) or lean protein
- ☐ Mixed greens, salad, or veggies
- ☐ Olive oil
- ☐ Apple cider vinegar

Totals for the day:

- Calories: 1,450
- Protein: 139g (~40%)
- Fat: 49g (~30%)
- Carbs: 114g (~30%)

FULL DAY OF EATING EXAMPLE: MEAL PLAN B–200 LB MALE

10 am—Breakfast

Protein + Fat, NO Starchy Carbs

- ☐ Veggie omelet or scrambled: 2 egg, 3 egg whites, veggies, non-stick spray
- ☐ 70%+ dark chocolate (1 serving)

Alternative breakfast strategy for when busy or traveling:

- ☐ 2 servings of protein powder (whey or egg) with water or almond milk (use blender or shaker cup), add greens powder, have with mixed nuts
- ☐ 70%+ dark chocolate (1 serving)

12 pm—Lunch

Protein + Carbs, Limit Fat

- ☐ 7 ounces of lean protein (chicken breast, tuna, cod, turkey breast, shrimp, white fish, etc.)
- ☐ 2 serving of healthy carbs (sweet potato, brown rice, quinoa, lentils, any kind of beans)
- ☐ Mixed veggies or spinach salad with light dressing

4 pm—Snack

Protein + Carbs, Limit Fat

- ☐ 2 serving of lean protein snack (organic beef jerky, tuna, or protein powder)
- ☐ 1 serving of steel cut oatmeal or fruit (berries, apple, orange, etc.)—can replace carbs with mixed nuts on non-training days

7 pm—Dinner

Protein + Fat, Limit Carbs

- ☐ 7 ounces of fattier protein (salmon, steak, lamb, pork) or lean protein
- ☐ Mixed greens, salad, or veggies
- ☐ Olive oil
- ☐ Apple cider vinegar

Totals for the day:

- Calories: 1,825
- Protein: 186g (~40%)
- Fat: 59g (~30%)
- Carbs: 139g (~30%)

APPROVED LIST OF FOODS TO MIX-AND-MATCH

Protein Options

- Eggs (any style; hard-boiled, scrambled, sunny side up, poached, fried, etc.)
- Chicken breast
- Trout (baked or seared)
- Mahi mahi (baked or pan seared)
- Pork (lean cuts only)
- Chicken tenders
- Shrimp (boiled, grilled or BBQ'd)
- Turkey burgers (grilled or seared)
- Ahi tuna steak (baked or pan seared)
- Turkey breast (grilled)
- Bison burger (leanest you can find)
- Steak (grass-fed where possible)

Carb Options (Are All Free of Gluten)

- Beans (any)
- Brown rice
- Quinoa
- Sweet potato
- Lentils
- Yucca (boiled)
- Plantains (boiled)
- Vegetable medley (or stir fry)
- Gluten free bread (toasted)

Snack Options: Protein

- Organic beef or bison jerky
- Smoked salmon jerky
- Boiled egg whites
- Vegetarian jerky
- Protein powder
- Hard-boiled eggs
- Yogurt
- Cheese

Snack Options: Carbs

- Granola bar (gluten free)
- Fruit (organic strawberry, blueberry, apples, oranges, etc.)
- Steel cut oatmeal
- Light butter popcorn
- Air popped chips

Snack Options: Healthy Fats

- Mixed Nuts (almonds, cashews, walnuts, hazelnut, etc).
- Seeds (chia, hemp, pumpkin, sunflower, etc.)
- Avocado

Notes:

- Feel free to mix and match these options to create variety
- Meals featuring single ingredients (e.g., chicken with broccoli and brown rice) are much easier to track and estimate macronutrients for than meals with combo ingredients (e.g., burrito, lasagna, etc.); stick to more single-ingredient type meals as much as possible.
- This list is not exhaustive. Feel free to add food to it as long as they meet the guidelines of *The Nine Shifts* nutrition strategy (e.g., are whole foods, low in gluten, low glycemic index/high fiber carbs, etc.).
- If you're not sure (e.g., "Can I have ketchup"?) just go back to nutrition guidelines and also gauge the impact of the calories and macronutrients to your overall targets.
- These meal plans represent what a typical eating strategy should look like. They are not customized to the individual. Adjustments may be required to match your specific situation. Please get in touch with us if you'd like support with this.

SHOPPING LIST

- Eggs—Large
- Broccoli
- Peppers, Mushrooms, Tomatoes, etc.
- Coconut Oil
- Whey or Egg Protein Powder
- Mixed Nuts
- Granola Bars
- Mixed Green Salad
- Olive Oil or Avocado Oil
- Apple Cider Vinegar (or Balsamic)
- Lean Protein (Chicken Breast, Turkey Breast, Tuna, etc.)
- Fattier Protein (Salmon, Steak, Pork, Lamb, etc.)
- Sweet Potato or Brown Rice or Quinoa or Any Beans or Lentil
- Mixed Veggies or Spinach Salad
- Light Dressing

Text this list to yourself to have handy when you shop!

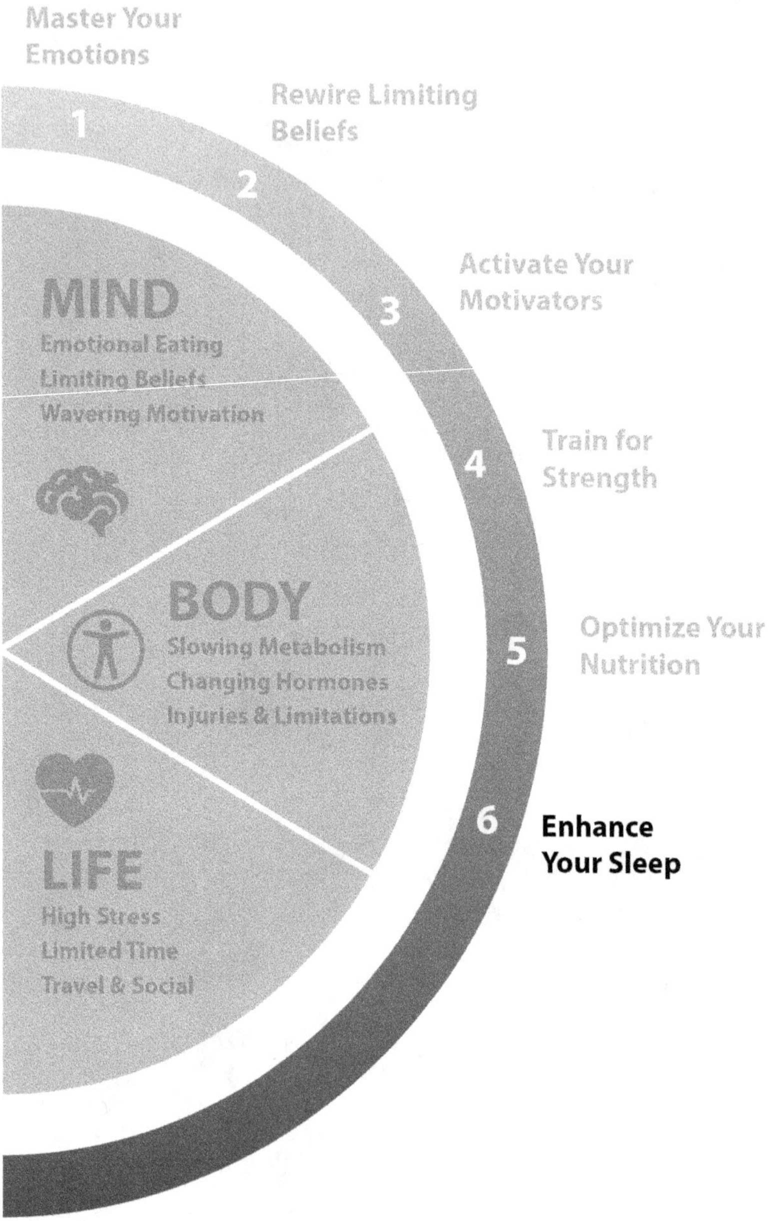

Master Your Emotions

1

Rewire Limiting Beliefs

2

Activate Your Motivators

3

MIND
Emotional Eating
Limiting Beliefs
Wavering Motivation

Train for Strength

4

BODY
Slowing Metabolism
Changing Hormones
Injuries & Limitations

Optimize Your Nutrition

5

6

Enhance Your Sleep

LIFE
High Stress
Limited Time
Travel & Social

CHAPTER 21

SHIFT #6: Enhance Your Sleep

"Sleep is the golden chain that binds
health and our bodies together."
—Thomas Dekker

Now, let's talk about an aspect of your body transformation journey that is much more important than most people may realize: getting your Z's.

Sleep is the third major input of your metabolism. Most people make mistakes in this area, including underestimating the importance of sleep, unknowingly depriving themselves of proper sleep, and not having any strategies or rituals to optimize their sleep. Indeed, it's estimated that 35% of U.S. adults do not get the recommended 7–8 hours of quality sleep per night.[61] In order get this step right, here is the key shift you will make:

KEY SHIFT

Go from insufficient, lower quality sleep to getting sufficient, higher quality rest and recovery.

When it comes to making a change in our body we've been conditioned to think about changing how we eat and exercise. I mean, how many times have we heard the worn out advice of *"Eat less and move more"*?

Optimizing sleep is an area that many over-40 professionals neglect.

With everyone focusing on diet and exercise, it's less intuitive to think about sleep (as well as the mindset transformation piece, as mentioned). However, this oversight doesn't make sleep any less important of a player in the game of transforming your body. In fact, Matthew Walker, a Harvard neuroscientist and author of the book *Why We Sleep: Unlocking The Power of Sleep and Dreams,*[62] calls sleep a key pillar of the "holy trinity of good health" (along with nutrition and exercise).

THE THREE PILLARS OF GOOD HEALTH

FOOD
FITNESS
SLEEP

There are several obstacles that make it hard to get our sleep right.

First, is the go-go, hustle culture of our times. In a global study of industrialized nations, 62% of adults reported that they undersleep.[63] Hustle culture creates constant pressure to be more and more productive at work. This creates a dynamic where the ability to work long hours on little sleep is seen as a badge of honor.

On top of this, professionals bring their job-related stress (and even their work) home with them, making it hard to wind down properly in order to get proper sleep.

The second obstacle to getting proper sleep is the always-on mode of being plugged into our devices. Our computers, tablets, and mobile phones are a source of constant distraction and temptation. The endless stream of notifications from social media, messaging apps, and email continuously suck our time, focus, and attention. It's been estimated that the working professional can get an average of almost 100 phone notifications per day.[64] Streaming services like Netflix lure us in with a constant flow of new, juicy shows and documentaries to binge on. Addictive video games keep us wanting to play longer and longer. These persistent disruptions and temptations can make it hard to unplug and sleep at an optimal hour.

The third obstacle is the mind's innate tendency to constantly worry, wonder, and ruminate. Ever have trouble falling asleep because you're worried you'll forget to pay an important bill the next day? Do you stay up (over-)analyzing an argument you had with a loved one? Have you tossed and turned in bed wondering whether you'll make it to the airport on time or not the next morning? Yup, these are all examples of our mind "doing its thing" and keeping us worried and awake.

Due to these factors, many over-40 professionals are perpetually underslept. Waking up tired, they down multiple cups of coffee to get them through their day. Because caffeine is a stimulant that creates alertness by blocking adenosine, a neurotransmitter that plays a key role in our sleep cycle, too much caffeine—especially too late in the day—robs us of proper sleep at night. In turn, we sleep poorly again, and feel "wired and tired" the next day. Waking up groggy, we reach for more of our favorite Colombian coffee blend. For many of us, this cycle continues throughout the workweek.

Whether you've struggled to sleep due to the factors above or you seem to sleep okay but are curious about how to enhance your sleep and recovery further, this chapter will act like a "wake up call" to the importance of sleep and will help you optimize this key area.

Furthermore, you'll be given a clear structure to follow via *The Nine Shifts* Sleep Enhancement Plan. It contains simple, science-based practices for optimizing your sleep. It's designed to help you recover properly from both your daily life and your training sessions. It includes a mix of strategies and rituals that ensure you get proper Zs and keep your metabolism in prime condition.

THE IMPORTANCE OF SLEEP

Sleep is essential for keeping us functioning well. During sleep our body performs essential duties, including repairing cells, rebuilding muscle lost during exercise, elevating your immune system to fight off intruders and diseases, priming brain function and cognition and restoring hormonal levels, including insulin, to their optimal state.

Conversely, when we don't sleep enough we get into what is known as sleep debt, which means sleeping fewer hours than what our body requires. Like with our credit cards, if we accumulate too much sleep debt, problems begin.

Poor sleep will slow your metabolism, while increasing inflammation and body fat. Other consequences of poor sleep include:

- elevated cortisol and blood sugar levels (since lack of sleep is a form of stress)
- hunger and cravings (due to ghrelin elevation)
- potential for overeating (due to less leptin sensitivity)
- gastrointestinal dysfunction (acid reflux, constipation, leaky gut, bloating, etc.)
- diminished sex hormone function including low T and menstrual irregularities
- impaired cognition and decision making (brain fog)
- emotional dysregulation (moodiness, depression, etc.)

Okay, so by this point, you're getting a sense of how important sleep actually is, and, after hearing all this, might be contemplating hopping into bed this very second to avoid all the havoc that might be coming your way if you sleep poorly again tonight.

The good news is that improving your sleep can quickly get you back on track and help you avoid the issues that come with poor sleep—almost overnight!

THE APPROACH

The main objective of your sleep approach will be to make sure you're consistently getting high quality sleep so you can recover from the stress of your day, the exertion of your workouts, and give your body a chance to do all the sleep-related functions that will keep you optimal.

To enhance our sleep, we must prioritize it and then optimize it.

First, you'll create the right sleep environment because things like temperature, noise, and even what you sleep on, all make a difference in the quality of the sleep you get. Second, you will adopt good sleep hygiene practices. These are habits that will ensure you're limiting the things that can disturb the quality of your sleep, such as eating or exposing yourself to blue light too close to bedtime. Third, you will properly prepare your body by managing stress at night via a proper wind-down routine. This will prevent elevating cortisol at night, which can make it hard to fall asleep and get quality rest.

In addition to the three principles above, be sure you are being mindful of, and addressing, any potential sleep disorders such as insomnia, obstructive sleep apnea, and snoring. On this last point, carrying excess weight that leads to the dreaded "double chin" can obstruct proper breathing during sleep, resulting in poor quality rest.

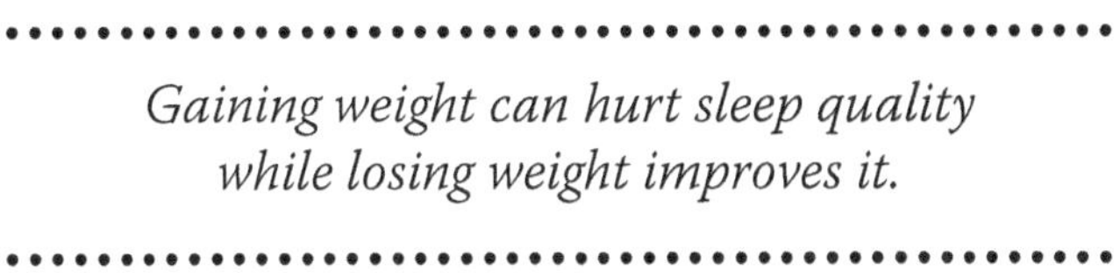

The good news is losing weight reverses this condition and helps us to sleep more deeply. In one study, there was an 83% reduction in the number of patients who reported snoring after losing weight, along with a 94% reduction in those suffering from sleep apnea.[65]

The Sleep Enhancement Plan will empower you with science-based strategies to improve your sleep and optimize this key, third pillar of boosting your metabolism (while priming your health and performance). Let's dive into the three key principles you will follow.

THE RIGHT SLEEP ENVIRONMENT

Our environment plays a key role in the quality of sleep we get. For starters, you want to make sure your room is dark. Melatonin is suppressed (and cortisol elevates) when our optic nerve perceives light. Dimming or blocking the lights on electronics in the bedroom, using black out shades to block external light, and using eye masks are all useful ways to ensure your room is sufficiently dark.

You also want to ensure that your sleeping space is quiet. Sounds can disturb your slumber, especially during the lighter phases of sleep. Make sure TVs, radios, and cell phones are silenced. Ideally, don't have them in your bedroom at all. Consider using earplugs or white noise to mask sounds. These tools are especially helpful if your partner snores (and using them is much less of a hassle than getting a divorce!).

Another aspect to consider is the temperature of your room. In short, your room must be cool enough. Our body temperature naturally drops as we move into sleep mode.[66] Being hot while trying to fall asleep can make things harder. This is actually a reason to not exercise too intensely late at night.

An additional factor to consider is movement, which can also be a sleep disruptor. Short of hip-checking your partner and sending them flying off the mattress and on to the floor for fidgeting too much in their sleep, there are some simple things you can do to limit unnecessary movements from affecting your Z's. For starters, I highly recommend not sleeping with pets; neither in the same bed nor the same bedroom. (Fido's gotta know that your bedroom is off-limits. Sorry, little guy.)

Similarly, it's best to not sleep with children, if possible. It's one thing if they're a newborn. But toddlers and infants may need some weaning off sleeping with mommy or daddy so they can act like "big kids" who sleep in their own crib or bed. This can help you get better Z's.

SLEEP HYGIENE PRACTICES

Below is a short list of what I feel are the best sleep hygiene habits to improve your Z's. (You'll find a longer list in the Sleep Enhancement Plan in this chapter.) Most of these habits are simple and cost nothing to do, so start using them as soon as tonight to improve your sleep quality.

Follow the 3-2-1 Rule

This rule makes it easy to remember some key wind-down habits that limit some of the main sleep disruptors: going to bed with a full stomach, waking up in the middle of the night to have to go pee, and being overstimulated by blue light close to bedtime.

The 3-2-1 Rule works like this:

- No food 3 hours before bed.
- No liquids 2 hours before bed.
- No screens 1 hour before bed.

Do all three above and watch how much more rested you feel the next morning.

Honor Your Body's Sleep-Wake Cycle

Going to bed at the same time (ideally, at a good time like 10pm or 11pm), and waking up at the same time is beneficial for optimizing your sleep schedule. This helps us work with, and not against, our body's circadian rhythm. For instance, the body shuts down digestion when we sleep, thus, eating too close to bedtime or in the middle of the night forces the body to digest food when it's not supposed to. Not only does this lead to poor digestion of said food, but also leads to poor sleep because digestion requires energy and forcing the body to digest food while sleeping means it can not process its sleep phases properly.

That being said, while we don't want to eat in the middle of the night or have a heavy meal too close to bedtime, we also don't want to skip dinner altogether. Remember the body likes things "just right," like Goldilocks. Having enough food at night, including having a small serving of healthy carbs, helps our nervous system relax.

Get Some Physical Activity during the Day

Get exercise, walking, or other physical activity during the day. This can help with falling asleep more easily at night. In fact, studies have found that proper exercise can help reduce sleep-related problems and improve the quality of rest you get during sleep.[67]

Even taking post-dinner walks, either outdoors or on a treadmill, helps with digestion and relaxation prior to bedtime. This can also better regulate blood sugar levels and keep body fat low, both of which help improve sleep quality.

WINDING DOWN PROPERLY

Most people don't have a strategy to transition properly into sleep, and no, passing out on the couch while watching TV doesn't count as a strategy. We want to be more mindful and take proactive steps to effectively switch over into the sleep phase of our day. When cortisol is chronically elevated at night time it limits melatonin production, and this hampers the quality of your sleep.

Thus, limiting cortisol at night by effectively managing stress and stimulation through a wind-down routine is a must if you want to sleep well. There are simple, hassle-free practices for managing stress in the evenings.

- Journaling about your day to release any negative thoughts or anxiety, and to celebrate your wins (no matter how small; my fellow high achievers, I'm looking at you!).
- Reviewing your to-do's list(s) and updating it to feel more grounded and ready for tomorrow.

- Closing your eyes, taking some deep breaths and giving gratitude (if you're inspired to do a full meditation, go for it; it can ease you into sleep).

> **Pro Tip:** One thing you can do to gauge how well you're sleeping is to use a sleep tracker like the Oura ring or the Rise app. These devices provide sleep data, like a daily sleep and recovery score, reveal sleep quality and sleeping patterns, and make suggestions for improving your sleep that's based on actual data versus just how you're feeling, which sometimes can be hard to use as a gauge for how well you've slept or not (especially after three cups of coffee).

THE SLEEP ENHANCEMENT PLAN

GUIDELINES:

- Time Required: Varies (depending on how many sleep tactics you will implement)
- What You Will Need: A pen, something to write on (optional: an Amazon account)
- Like with the other habits in *The Nine Shifts*, start small and do what's easy initially so you can feel successful and avoid any resistance from the mind's comfort zone to daunting tasks or goals.
- Some of the items are free or low-cost to incorporate (e.g., gratitude, journaling, blue light glasses, sleep

supplements, etc.) Others require more of an investment (e.g., quality mattress, sleep tracking device). Use or get whichever tools or tactics feel right to you.

STEPS:

- ☐ Create the right sleep environment
- ☐ Follow good sleep hygiene practices
- ☐ Wind down properly

STEP #1: CREATE THE RIGHT SLEEP ENVIRONMENT

Here are some ways to ensure your environment is set up for optimal sleep:

- dark room (use "the hand test"; shouldn't be able to see your palm in the dark)
- cool room (use air conditioning, fans, etc., as needed)
- silent room (block out external noises with a white noise machine or app)
- disturbance-free room; no "little visitors" (do not sleep with children if possible; do not allow pets in bedroom)

STEP #2: FOLLOW GOOD SLEEP HYGIENE PRACTICES

- Follow the 3-2-1 rule. No eating 3 hours before bed, no drinking 2 hours before bed, no screens 1 hour before bed.
- Honor Sleep-Wake cycles (go to bed and wake up at the same time; sun exposure in AM).

- Get physical activity during the day (walks and imperfect actions help with this).
- Avoid too much caffeine, especially in the afternoon after 3PM (coffee, tea, chocolate, energy drinks, etc.).
- Limit alcohol consumption as alcohol compromises sleep quality.
- Use blue light blocking glasses when viewing screens at night, blue light suppresses production of melatonin.
- Limit intense exercise or working late at night before bed to limit cortisol at night.
- Have a small serving of healthy carbs in your last meal (carbs suppress cortisol and help us relax).

STEP #3: WIND DOWN PROPERLY

Some ways to wind down and transition properly into sleep are below. Write down a few that feel good to you and start implementing them tonight!

- Limit working, exercising intensely, engaging in controversial topics, or other stimulation too late in the evening (schedule a time for it the next day).
- Give gratitude (helps to ease stress and anxiety immediately).
- Journal your day (celebrate three wins, dump out any stress or negative emotion on to the paper, jot down any to do's, plan your next day's intention and important tasks).
- Light stretching and movement (helps calm the mind and creates a positive emotional state).

- Meditate and be mindful (helps bring down the autonomic nervous system to allow good rest; you can use guided meditations found on Youtube or meditation apps).
- Avoid the temptation to check your phone right before bed (or first thing upon waking); especially NOT while in bed!

Pro Tip: On this last point, not checking your phone last thing before bed or first thing when you wake up helps avoid distractions, allowing you to start and end your day grounded and in control.

You just fully completed this chapter.

Keep going and keep your transformation moving forward!

CHAPTER 22

Momentum 101

"Each morning we are born again. What we do today is what matters most."
—Buddha

Alright! Another virtual high five is in order. I want to take a moment and say "great work!" By enthusiastically taking on the last section, Metabolism, you've ensured that age-related challenges of a slowing metabolism, changing hormones, and the potential for injuries do not get in the way of your desired body and health. (Whoop!)

Because you've now addressed both the Mindset and the Metabolism parts of the *Nine Shifts*, you've made sure mental challenges will not get in your way, and you know which metabolism-boosting habits to keep—around training, nutrition, and sleep—to make your body lean, strong, healthy, and energized.

Now, let's make sure your body will stay that way.

How?

By preventing life's challenges from derailing your consistency.

HOW THIS PART OF THE BOOK KEEPS YOUR BODY WHERE YOU WANT IT

The Momentum part of the *Nine Shifts* body transformation framework will guide you to make three key shifts that will prevent external obstacles from ruining your body progress:

1. Mitigate External Stressors
2. Keep Efficient Habits
3. Navigate Travel & Social Events

These three shifts will empower you to overcome the challenges brought on by our external environment: high stress, limited time, and travel & social events. By making these three shifts, we will side-step these life-related challenges, stay consistent, and maintain our transformed body for good.

The three chapters that follow will share proven strategies and steps for handling things life will throw at you, including stress from getting triggered by people, not having enough time in the day, and the temptations of eating poorly when traveling or at social events.

You will learn practices for getting grounded and creating a shield against external stress, for creating time and space to do your habits efficiently each week, and for preparing before travel and events so you don't get thrown off your routine. Ultimately, you will learn how to keep your hard-earned results by harnessing the power of momentum.

Without this piece, all of the energy, time, and focus you'll put into empowering your mind and elevating your metabolism will go to waste. Needless to say, your ability to stay consistent is essential to keeping your body results for a lifetime.

Ask anyone who got in shape but fell off, or lost weight but then regained it; they'll tell you that maintaining your results is a lot harder than attaining them. You've probably experienced this yourself in your own health journey. Regardless, I'm sure you'll agree that there's nothing worse than doing what it takes to achieve results, only to lose them and have to start all over. Whether we're talking about working hard to make a lot of money and losing it all, or losing weight but having it come back, it's an awful situation.

Unfortunately, this is what a lot of people have to deal with. As mentioned, 90% of dieters gain back all of the weight they lost during their diet, if not more.

But that's not going to be you.

WHY "CONSISTENCY IS KEY" IS BS

The next time someone preaches to you that "consistency is key," please take this book—or the device you're reading it on—and proceed to slap them across the face with it; hard. (It's ok, you can blame it on me.)

They don't deserve the slap because consistency is not important (it is) or because they're stating the obvious (no duh!). They deserve it because preaching to someone that consistency is key has never made anyone more consistent.

The only way to get more consistent, and keep your transformed body for life, is to navigate both the internal and external challenges that can kill your consistency. These are the nine most common challenges we talked about in Part II of the book.

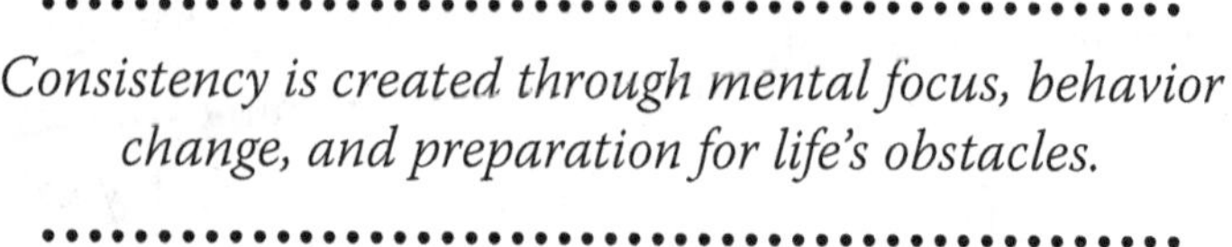

Consistency is created through mental focus, behavior change, and preparation for life's obstacles.

This is much easier said than done.

Most people will fail and regress.

It's why the majority of the people in the United States stay overweight or obese. It's why marketers try to sell us weight loss powders, fat loss injections, and testosterone replacement therapy. It's why heart disease and diabetes, as well as mental health disorders, are at historic highs. It's why big and beautiful stores exist and why the internet is abuzz with the hashtag #fatshaming.

People have become forlorn. After all the back and forth between making progress, then relapsing, they've become hopeless. Attaining the body and health they once had feels impossible.

Mind you, I'm not saying any of this is bad, nor am I passing judgment in any way. I am saying it's not optimal and has created a sad state of affairs that we have to resort to overhyped products, shortcuts, and false promises.

But all is not bleak.

THE GOOD NEWS FOR YOU (THINGS ARE ABOUT TO GET EASIER)

By getting to this point in the book, you've actually done a lot of the heavy lifting—no pun intended! Let me quickly say: "Thank you for hanging in there!"

You've now gotten through the most complex aspects of achieving a permanent body transformation. You've learned about the psychology of the mind and the science of the body. Now, all that's left is to gain the skill of maintaining your momentum.

This next part of the book will feel easy-breezy. It will also be the shortest part of the three parts of *The Nine Shifts* framework.

But do yourself a favor and do ***not*** underestimate the importance of this next part.

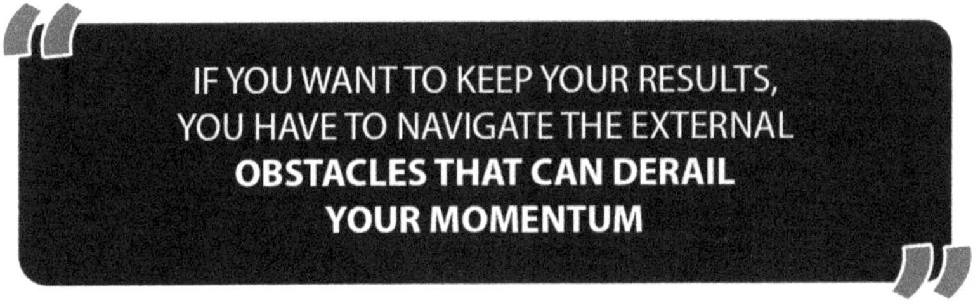

If you don't learn the strategies that will help overcome the external obstacles from throwing you off, I can't promise that you will hold on to the changes you make in your body by executing the mindset and metabolism parts of this book.

The curveballs from work and life are out there, and they're waiting for you.

HOW MOMENTUM, MINDSET, AND METABOLISM ARE CONNECTED

This part of the book makes a perfect capstone to what you've learned so far. There is a tight interdependency between the habits we need to perform for our mind and our body with our ability to stay on track with those habits.

- From a **mindset** standpoint, we know it's important to minimize the impact of stress, not get burnt out by overcompensating for our deep-seated fears, and keeping our motivation high.
- From a **body** standpoint, we have to do the right things from a training, eating, and sleeping perspective to keep our metabolism elevated. In order to do that, we have to make sure mental challenges like stress and overcompensation don't kill our motivation.
- From a **momentum** standpoint, we have to make sure life and work demands don't result in too much internal stress that can affect the body (our physiology) or kill our motivation (our psychology). We also have to make sure these outside forces don't result in robbing us of our time and ability to do the training, eating, and sleeping we need to do to keep our body where it needs to be.

Simply put, letting outside forces hurt our momentum will result in reduced motivation and will prevent us from doing what it takes to keep our metabolism elevated.

A HIGH-LEVEL OVERVIEW OF MOMENTUM

In 1686, British mathematician Sir Isaac Newton discovered the Law of Motion. It says, "A body in motion at a constant velocity will remain in motion in a straight line unless acted upon by an outside force."

That's a perfect analogy for this chapter (thanks Izzy!). The operative words here are "outside force." It's those outside forces that can knock you off your trajectory that I want you to be prepared for.

We want to make sure that things like not having enough time, being tempted by outside foods, or having to travel will not deprive you of the health and body you worked so hard for. You'll learn:

- How to increase your chances of staying consistent with best practices around weekly scheduling.
- How to set the right boundaries with the people in your life to create the "space" needed for your ongoing self-care. (Yes, people pleasers, even you!)
- How to perform your body transformation habits quickly so they don't require you to sacrifice precious time for the people and things you love.
- How to minimize the damage from social events that involve rich foods and alcohol, such as weddings, birthdays, Thanksgiving and other holidays, while still enjoying them.
- How to prepare for trips so that food at airports and truck stops don't derail your progress.

In addition, I'll do my best to prepare you for the most common curveballs that I see my clients struggle with, including work deadlines, client events, and family obligations.

THE LINK BETWEEN MOMENTUM AND MOTIVATION

You can say that momentum and motivation are bedfellows. You really can't have one without the other. Motivation creates momentum and momentum makes you feel motivated. When one goes up the other goes up with it.

Conversely, when one goes down the other is sure to follow.

The main difference is that motivation is something you feel, whereas momentum is esoteric; it's more of a concept or an ideal.

The good news is that you've already been given a solid game plan for how to keep your motivation from wavering, in Chapter 17, "Shift #3: Activate Your Motivators." If you follow those strategies, you will give yourself a great shot at maintaining your momentum. Unless, of course, someone or something gets in your way.

Like with motivation, the airplane analogy also applies here. It takes a lot more fuel to get your momentum off the ground if it's sitting there like a plane in a hangar, than it does to keep cruising along at altitude. Similar to motivation, we want to have tiny peaks and valleys in our momentum, and make small adjustments and course corrections so that it doesn't nosedive.

THE GOAL IS NOT TO BE PERFECT

Now, I realize that pretty much no one has the ability to always be consistent no matter what happens. We all deal with challenges, stress, and things that need our attention.

I certainly don't expect someone dealing with demanding situations like moving their home, grieving a loss, or tending to a newborn or sick parent to be perfect with their routine.

The goal here is not to try to be perfect. The goal is to do our best to limit outside obstacles from setting us back too much, for too long.

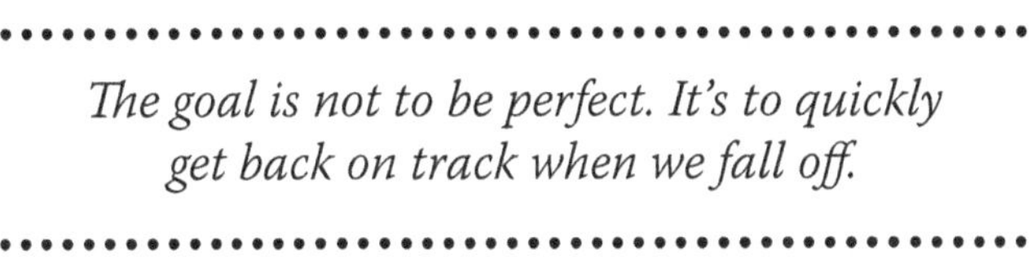
The goal is not to be perfect. It's to quickly get back on track when we fall off.

For the times we get knocked off track, the goal is to:

- Know where the track is, instead of having to guess at what to do.
- Get back to it smartly and quickly so you don't get stuck for long.

This book provides the blueprint for the track that will get you to your goal. It helps you know what adjustments to make in your mindset, fitness, and meals in order to start making progress again.

It also provides you with tactics and strategies for minimizing the damage of outside disruptions, and helps you get back on track quickly so that obstacles—big or small—don't derail you for too long. (And yes, I realize you're not a train, or a plane, but I think you get my point.)

LET'S TACKLE THE THREE MAIN WAYS THAT LIFE PREVENTS YOUR BODY TRANSFORMATION

Now that you have a better understanding of how your mind and body operate, there are three main ways life can interfere with your body transformation. Here they are below, with the corresponding chapter that will address it.

EXTERNAL STRESSORS CAUSE INTERNAL STRESS

Many people fall prey to outside distractions or get triggered by what goes on around them. This includes getting triggered by other people. These external stressors can cause internal stress and cause us to break consistency with our body transformation habits.

To empower you in these situations, you will learn simple-but-powerful morning and evening routines that will empower you to start and end your day on a powerful note. They will enable you to create a shield for the distractions and stress caused by external forces so you can stay in momentum with your body transformation habits.

We will tackle this in Chapter 23, "Shift #7: Mitigate External Stressors."

INEFFICIENT HABITS CAN CAUSE US TO QUIT DOING THEM

If our body transformation routine takes too long and starts feeling like a second job, we have little chance of sustaining it over the long run.

To give you the best chance of staying in momentum, you will learn how to get your routine done in minimal time—just 3–5 hours per week. Better yet, it will show you how to do it in a way that's flexible and works with your schedule.

We will cover this in Chapter 24, "Shift #8: Keep Efficient Habits."

TRAVEL AND SOCIAL EVENTS POSE CHALLENGES TO OUR BODY

Traveling to other cities for work, making housecalls, seeing clients, or going on vacations create challenges that can knock us off of our routine. Similarly, having to attend social events full of rich food, and peer pressure to consume them, can also set us back from progress we've made in our body.

I will help you prepare for, and effectively navigate, these scenarios so that they don't set you back, cause demotivation, and thwart your momentum.

We will tackle this in Chapter 25, "Shift #9: Navigate Travel & Social Events."

As you can see, maintaining our momentum is essential.

So let's keep going!

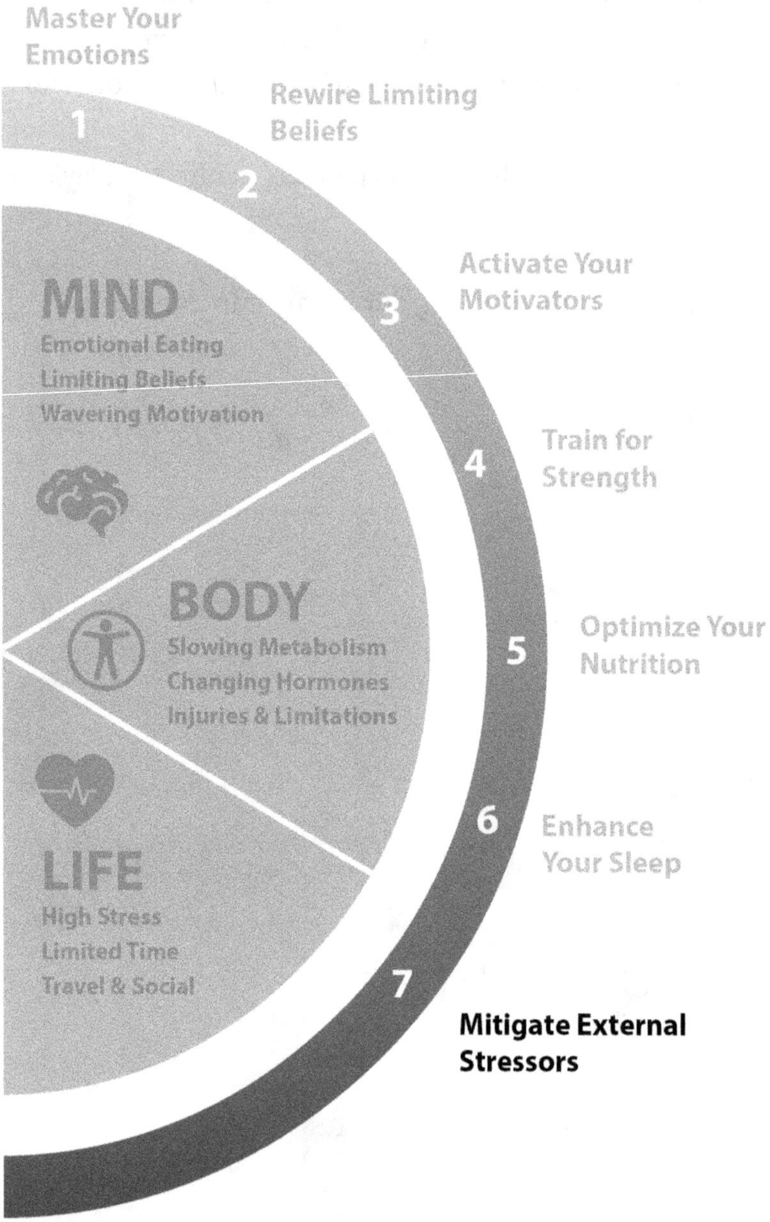

Master Your Emotions

1

Rewire Limiting Beliefs

2

Activate Your Motivators

3

MIND

Emotional Eating
Limiting Beliefs
Wavering Motivation

Train for Strength

4

BODY

Slowing Metabolism
Changing Hormones
Injuries & Limitations

Optimize Your Nutrition

5

Enhance Your Sleep

6

LIFE

High Stress
Limited Time
Travel & Social

7

Mitigate External Stressors

CHAPTER 23

SHIFT #7: Mitigate External Stressors

"Avoiding your triggers isn't healing. Healing happens when you're triggered and you're able to move through the pain, the pattern, and the story—and walk your way to a different ending."
—Vienna Pharaon

Momentum upgrade loading . . .

Now, let's cover the first aspect of maintaining our momentum: mitigating external stress.

Many people fall prey to outside distractions or get triggered by what goes on around them. This includes getting triggered by other people. In fact, it seems that people are generally angrier and get more triggered these days. In a poll by NPR, 84% of participants felt that Americans are angrier compared to a generation ago.[68]

When we get triggered by external stressors, it can cause internal stress, which, in turn, can cause us to break consistency with our body transformation habits (e.g., emotional eating, skipping workouts, etc.). But that won't be you because you're about to learn how to make this key shift:

KEY SHIFT

Go from reacting to what the world throws at you to being in control and responding from a place of power.

This shift will empower you to not get derailed by outside forces that are out of your control and greatly improve your chances of keeping that hard-earned body over a lifetime. You will learn how to do this by going through this chapter and completing the External Stress Mitigation Plan that's coming up soon.

THE APPROACH

As with mastering your emotions and maintaining your motivation, the goal here is to perform simple daily practices that will keep you grounded and in a positive emotional state. No matter what the day hurls your way, you will be calm and in control instead of reactionary or stressed out.

Starting and ending the day calm and in control makes us less reactionary to the outside world. This, in turn, helps us maintain our habits and our momentum.

Executing the steps in the External Stress Mitigation Plan will help change your relationship with external stressors from one where you have no strategy for protecting your time, attention, and emotions from outside events, and get easily distracted or triggered, to one where external stress is something you are taking control over.

Instead of just going with the flow like most people do and getting thrown for a loop when life hits them with something stressful, you will proactively put yourself in a more empowered state to handle curveballs better than 99% of folks.

My client, Nick, the investment banker you met, who deals with intense confrontations during his negotiations at work, said, "The strategies in the plan helped me to be more grounded. I have a month of meetings coming up for a new client and I feel more confident going into those now." Indeed, they can also empower you to feel more confident going into any challenging conversation or situation you might have to face.

Let's dive into the three key practices to follow.

DAILY EMPOWERMENT ROUTINE (MORNING AND EVENING)

To truly create a shield from external stressors, having a daily empowerment routine is essential. It allows you to be intentional about how your day will go versus just going into your day unconsciously and hoping for the best. It will also elevate your metabolism, energy, and inner strength, preparing you for whatever the day throws at you.

Yet, very few people have practices to start their day in a powerful way. As a case in point, 80% of Americans check their phone within fifteen minutes of waking up in the morning. (Not optimal.)[69]

This can cause us to begin our day in a reactionary mode, feeling overwhelmed or anxious upon seeing the numerous emails, notifications, and other messages coming at us before we even get a chance to set our focus on what's most important to accomplish in the day ahead.

When it comes to our evening rituals they usually aren't much better. According to The Sleep Foundation, "95 percent of Americans watch some kind of content on a screen in the hour before bed."[70] (Confession: I'm guilty of doing this myself.)

This robs us of an opportunity to reflect back on our day and to start preparing for the next one. But having an evening ritual is essential for completing your day and releasing any stress that may have accumulated during the day. Taking time to wind down properly helps you with optimizing sleep (which, as you know, is essential for your metabolism, health, and performance).

Keeping this type of nightly routine means shifting from entertainment at night to more introspection. But it's worth it because ending your day victoriously in this way helps you start the next day in control and way more ready for life's stressors.

PEAK STATE RITUAL

Putting yourself in what's known as a peak state (or peak emotional state) is one of the secrets of overall life success. Not only will it help you fend off external stressors, it will greatly improve your outcomes at everything you do.

You can think about it this way—which version of you has a greater chance of succeeding at life?

A. The version of you that is average to below average in energy, confidence, strength, and clarity?

B. The version of you that is your most energized, confident, strong, and clear?

The obvious answer is version B. Thus, to be successful, we want to be putting ourselves in a peak state as much as possible. We can do this through rituals and routines.

It's similar to how an athlete goes through their pre-game habits and warm-ups. They're preparing themselves to perform by getting their body moving, their energy up, and focusing their mind. They visualize what they will do on the field or court when it's time to execute. These rituals put their body in a peak physical and emotional state, and allow them to unlock a peak mental state (also known as a "state of flow") where things become effortless. Ultimately, these rituals give them the confidence and preparation needed to play their best.

In the same way, you want to start preparing yourself to play your best every day. Part of the goal of your morning routine will be to put yourself in a peak state and prepare you to perform your best. Remember, the version of you that is most empowered, energized, confident, and focused has the best chance of succeeding in whatever you're up to—as well as creating immunity against external stressors.

You can also come up with some small go-to rituals you can quickly perform to put yourself in a peak state before important conversations, meetings, and presentations so you can be more grounded and exude confidence.

RESPONDING VERSUS REACTING (AND THE RECREATING TECHNIQUE)

The key to not getting triggered is to respond from a place of control versus reacting from a place of fear or defensiveness. When we react, it's an emotional response and logic goes out the window. This leads to poor outcomes.

The trick is to be more aware of how the ego can take over and cause us to say something or retaliate without much thought. This often happens in conversations. A powerful technique that will help you respond and not react when it comes to potentially getting triggered by others is the recreating technique.

The Recreating Technique

This technique provides you with personal power to not let what others say affect you negatively. Developing this skill goes beyond the cliched outcome of "developing thicker skin," which is mostly about ignoring the other person and comes from ego. This creates distance and resentment.

In the process of recreating, you leave the person feeling heard and honored. Recreating creates understanding and partnership, but also sets a boundary where it's needed.

You gain the ability to be in any conversation, with anyone.

We will do a quick role play in Step #3 below so you can see how it works.

THE EXTERNAL STRESS MITIGATION PLAN

GUIDELINES:

- Time Required: 15–20 minutes
- What You Will Need: A pen, something to write on, and a quiet area

- Keep in mind that these techniques, when done correctly, give you the power to transform your relationships and your life by creating a shield around you from external forces that can trigger you.
- But like anything else worth having, it takes practice, practice, practice!

STEPS:

- ☐ Establish your morning and evening routine
- ☐ Keep your peak state ritual handy
- ☐ Practice the recreating technique

STEP #1: ESTABLISH YOUR DAILY EMPOWERMENT ROUTINE (MORNING & EVENING)

Step #1a. Morning Routine

To set an empowering context for your day, you want to practice an efficient routine every morning that gets your body moving a bit, your thoughts positive, and your focus on the present moment.

In order to do this, you will perform a combination of mindset and movement-related activities to get grounded and focused, and to get your blood flowing and your metabolism going. The goal is to generate a positive internal state.

Mindset activities can and should include some of the following:

- meditation
- journaling
- giving gratitude

- reconnecting with your "why" or InPowerment Word for transforming your body (e.g., "confidence")
- reconnecting with your new identity and future vision
- reciting affirmations that support your goals (e.g., "I stay healthy and strong to be there for my loved ones.")
- visualizing yourself moving closer to your goals
- creating context for who you will "be" today (e.g., "Today I get to be calm and happy.")

Movement activities can include:

- calisthenics and moving the body (light squats, jumping jacks)
- stretching and yoga poses
- power breathing or belly breaths
- a few minutes of jumping jacks or jumping rope (if your knees can take it)
- some squats (or half squat to chair)
- walking or a workout (if you choose)

Step #1b. Evening Routine

The goal of your evening routine is to properly wind you down and help you complete the day in a powerful way. One of the most important aspects of your evening routine is to create calm and shift your nervous system from sympathetic (fight or flight) to parasympathetic (rest and digest) mode. This is particularly important if you exercise in the evening. Downshifting your nervous system properly will allow you to sleep and recover optimally.

A big area to focus on is to not carry emotionally charged thoughts into bed as they may make it hard to fall asleep.

Your evening routine can and should include some of the following:

- reflecting back on the day
- celebrating wins, no matter how small
- giving gratitude
- journaling
- listening to calming music or a positive podcast or audiobook
- light stretching
- warm bath or shower
- drinking calming tea (caffeine free)
- planning for the next day
- handling quick loose ends
- having a loving chat
- reading or doing something relaxing that is device-free
- doing your sleep hygiene practices (from the Sleep Enhancement Plan in Chapter 21)

STEP #2: KEEP YOUR PEAK STATE RITUAL HANDY

The items mentioned in the morning ritual above work great for grounding you. But to really amp up your energy and focus before performing, you have to move energy through you. This means literally moving energy through your body by putting yourself in motion. Motion creates positive emotion. Thus, we want to move our bodies to start driving the energy up, nudging up the heart rate a bit, and get our body to be more focused. Times like these are when we want to purposely put ourselves in more of a fight or flight mode. This is where we are more alert, focused, and ready for action.

This doesn't mean doing a full workout. Just some empowering movements that are quick and practical to do.

For instance, before I have an important Zoom call or meeting, you'll usually find me doing some body weight squats or jumping jacks to get some positive emotion and energy flowing. I'll also state aloud an affirmation or state an intention for how I want the call or meeting to go.

The more energy and focus you bring, the more present, confident, and successful you will be. Plus, you'll be less susceptible to getting triggered or having outside forces throwing you off during said meeting or conversation. This includes preventing your core limiting belief from getting triggered if things don't go your way during your conversation or meeting.

Think about some things you can do right before you need to "perform" to put yourself in a peak state (e.g., do some squats, shake your body out, power breathing, jumping jacks, etc.). Write them down so you can have them handy the next time you need to be "on!"

STEP #3. PRACTICE THE RECREATING TECHNIQUE (ROLE PLAY EXERCISE)

The Old Way: Reacting to What's Being Said (Defending)

Visualize that you're about to go into a tense conversation that could potentially trigger you. Perhaps it's with a coworker, boss, client, or loved one. If it's easier, you can think of someone who has gotten under your skin before by teasing you, taking a jab at you, giving you an underhanded remark, or being passive aggressive.

For example, let's say a coworker is critical of something you did and says, "You idiot! You did a terrible job on that report! What's wrong with you?!"

Close your eyes and think about what thoughts and feelings just came up for you.

You most likely felt tension in your body and your mind went into a defensive or worried mode, right? These sensations are normal.

When we get a criticism the mind makes the words "mean" something about us. This negative meaning triggers our fears of not being good enough. The mind will always seek to defend you from criticism and looking bad.

When we do defend, what happens? The other person tries to make their case more emphatically. In turn, we defend more strongly. They continue trying to make their case and we continue trying to defend, and so on. From here, things can either escalate (not good) or if one party backs down, the other party feels unheard and this creates a rift or incompletion in the relationship.

The New Way: Being with What Is Said (Recreating)

Now, imagine if instead of reacting to what's being said, you simply absorb what's being said.

When you are "recreating" the other person, you're basically saying back to them exactly what they said to you, WITHOUT adding anything to it.

It will be tempting to add your own interpretation or counter-argument. That's because the mind is always on the lookout to defend you and anything it associates with being you (including your character, your identity, and your beliefs).

You are proactively looking out for the mind's tendency to add meaning to things and to defend, and releasing them. Then, you're saying back to the other person exactly what they said, without adding any meaning or emotion to it.

This diffuses any negative emotions that may come up in a conversation and prevents you from getting triggered.

So, when your coworker says: "You idiot! You did a terrible job on that report! What's wrong with you?!", you simply say back to him or her what you just heard, without making it about you, or them.

You can say something like: "So let me make sure I understood you correctly. You feel that I did a terrible job with that report and that you think I'm an idiot. Did I get that right?"

(If you feel a bit like a robot when you're saying their words back to them, you're doing it right!)

The beauty of "recreating" what they said in this way is that you disarm the other person. Once they feel (fully) heard, they know that their point was made and will no longer be in attack mode.

You can disarm them further by replying with empathy. You can start with understanding how they're feeling.

"I'm sorry that you feel I did a terrible job and that it made you upset."

Now, they'll feel you've totally "got" what they were trying to say.

This creates the space for you to explain your side, without coming from a place of defensiveness or attacking them back. They'll be more open to hearing your side, now that you've heard their side.

This is a powerful tool that leaves both parties heard and working in partnership towards a resolution instead of attacking and defending from their own point of view, which only leads to tension, mistrust, and hurt feelings.

I've used this technique to coach my clients through numerous difficult conversations in work settings and beyond. When done right, it can totally change your relationship dynamic with others and give you much more influence and power in your interpersonal relationships.

Mastering this technique will take practice because your mind will try to jump in and defend, every time. But over time, you'll be able to bring a grounded, cool, and empowered demeanor to your conversations, which will go a long way to ensuring successful relationships in your life.

It will also limit the potential for getting triggered, stressed, or demotivated so you can stay on track with your body transformation goals and keep your momentum going!

You just fully completed this chapter and now have a "shield" against external stress. Awesome!

Keep going and keep your transformation moving forward!

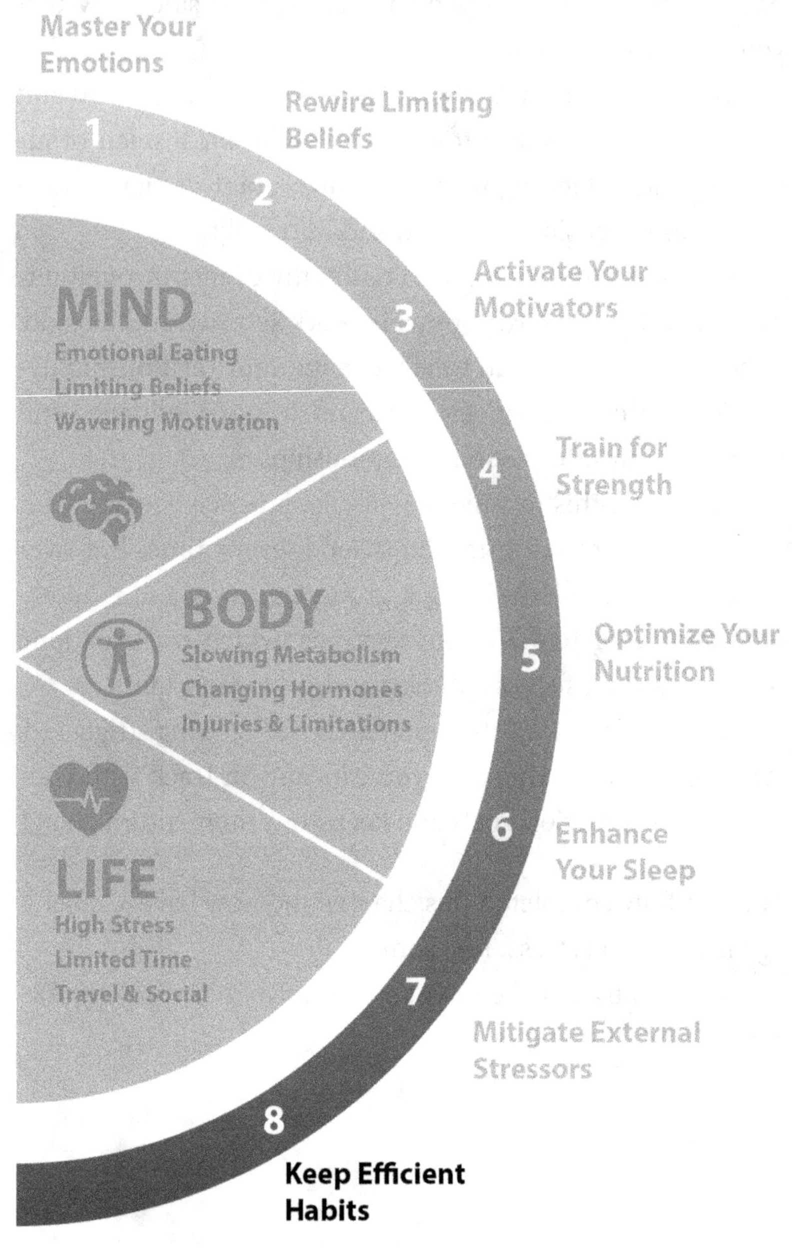
Master Your
Emotions
1
Rewire Limiting
Beliefs
2
MIND
Emotional Eating
Limiting Beliefs
Wavering Motivation
3
Activate Your
Motivators
4
Train for
Strength
BODY
Slowing Metabolism
Changing Hormones
Injuries & Limitations
5
Optimize Your
Nutrition
6
Enhance
Your Sleep
LIFE
High Stress
Limited Time
Travel & Social
7
Mitigate External
Stressors
8
Keep Efficient
Habits

CHAPTER 24

SHIFT #8: Keep Efficient Habits

"No such thing as spare time, no such thing as free time, no such thing as down time. All you got is life time. Go."
—Henry Rollins

Alright. Now we get to talk about one of my favorite topics: saving time. I'm assuming you agree that life is short and time is the most precious commodity we're given.

I'm also guessing that you have lots of things pulling at your time and that it's often hard to find spare time for yourself and your body transformation habits.

Finding the time to work out, eat proper meals, sleep sufficiently, and do mindset or self-care practices is a common struggle. In one survey, 60% of Americans said they didn't have enough time in the day to get all their work, chores, and errands done, and would love an additional four hours in the day to accomplish them all.[71] (Wouldn't that be amazing?!)

Despite their (perceived) time crunch, very few of these folks have a strategy to maximize their limited time. In order to make the most of the time you invest in your ongoing habits, here is the key shift you will make:

KEY SHIFT

Go from leaving your habits to chance or spending too much time for limited results, to proactively managing and doing the most effective habits efficiently and consistently.

This chapter will make sure that the challenge of not having enough time will never stop you again from attaining the body, confidence, and health you're after. You will learn how to do this by going through this chapter and completing the the Efficient Habits Implementation Plan that's coming up soon.

THE APPROACH

The main objective of the Efficient Habits Implementation Plan is to maximize your limited time and ensure, from a logistics standpoint, that you're doing your mind and body transformation habits consistently. If we break down this shift, you can see that it's made up of two parts: efficient and implementation. This means we have to keep our habits simple, make sure they deliver maximum results for the time we're spending, and have a process to make sure they get done.

Interestingly, these two objectives feed off of each other. If our habits are efficient, we'll be more likely to do them, allowing us to implement them and maintain our consistency.

Our habits need to be smart, simple, and scheduled, or they won't get done.

Taking this approach improves our consistency and keeps us in momentum. This is exactly what the Efficient Habits Implementation Plan will help you accomplish.

Executing the steps in the plan will help change your relationship with time from one where we struggle to find time to do our habits and feel overwhelmed, to one where we perform our habits consistently in minimal time per week, while getting the most ROI on our time spent.

Instead of just buying into the notion that "I don't have enough time" like most people do, you will proactively know what to do each week and fit your mind and body transformation habits easily into your schedule and into your life.

Not letting a busy schedule stop us from attaining and maintaining our desired body comes down to fitting our habits in on an ongoing basis. The more efficient they are, and the more proactively we plan them, the more we improve our chances of having the mind, body, and life we seek, through our golden age.

My client, Ron, who is 58 years old, had this to say about the Efficient Habits Implementation Plan: "I used to spend so much time each week trying to keep my body in a good place. But now, I do what I need to do more quickly and then go about my day. This has given me more time to spend on other things, like doing things with my family."

MAXIMIZE YOUR LIMITED TIME (PRIORITIZE THE 80/20)

While all of the habits you've been learning about in this book are important for attaining and maintaining your desired body, not all of these habits are created equal. Some will give you more bang for your buck. We have to focus on the 20% of habits that will give us 80% of our results. Below are what I consider the Top-5 "high value" habits for transforming your body. These are the ones you want to prioritize. If you do nothing else, make sure you do these each week:

1. **Meal prep religiously**—Meal prepping regularly is the one habit that gives you the best shot at keeping your body in a healthy, well functioning place. Nutrition alone won't make you optimal (for that you need the other habits in *The Nine Shifts*). But eating clean foods regularly as a result of regular meal prep can ensure you keep your body and health fairly close to where you want them to be.
2. **Strength train often**—Adds lean muscle, elevates your resting metabolic rate, and creates the after burn effect, which boosts your calorie burn for many hours after your workout is over.
3. **Stay connected to your "why"**—The mind is easily distracted. It forgets why this matters to you, and it prefers that you don't exert yourself. Staying connected to "why" being your fittest and best matters to you, and why it's a must for you to achieve it—at an identity level—will create urgency (which most people lack). This helps get you out of your comfort zone

and keeps you motivated to overcome the obstacles to consistency, like not having enough time!

4. **Take imperfect actions**—By being quick and easy to do, they help beat perfectionism, halt procrastination, create positive emotion, and sustain motivation.
5. **Set anchors & boundaries**—A crazy schedule makes it essential to literally schedule our habits into our calendar and create the freedom and space, through boundaries, to execute them at our set times. Otherwise, we leave our habits—and the body we desire—to chance. (More on this soon.)

ALWAYS SCHEDULE IT IN (USING ANCHORS)

They say that the road to hell is paved with good intentions. This is pretty apropos for body transformation.

Lots of people set out to do certain things during the week, such as exercise, go for a hike, prepare some healthy meals, take their supplements, or get good sleep. But when the week is over, they look back and realize they did very few, if any, of those things.

One of the biggest reasons is because they never had them in their schedule.

Many over-40 professionals miss doing their habits simply because they don't have them scheduled in their calendar.

You know the famous line from the movie *Glengarry Glen Ross* where the hot shot salesman role played by Alec

Baldwin preaches to the other salespeople "Always be closing."? Well, for us to be successful with our habits you want to "Always be scheduling."

Otherwise, we leave our consistency to chance. To prevent that from happening, we have to make time for our body transformation habits in a very literal sense; by blocking off the time in our calendar so that it's not just floating around in our head with the seven million other things you need to worry about.

I call these time blocks "anchors." As the name implies, they lock down time in your schedule to execute your activities. They also prevent others from double-booking you during those times. Just like a real anchor, they should hold strong in the face of life's currents, and they should not be moved except for rare exceptions and with great hesitation.

Best practices for setting your anchors, include making them automatically repeat each week and showing as "busy" to others (preventing them from double-booking you during those times).

If something important comes up during your scheduled weekly habit at the anchor time you've set, make sure you don't delete it. Instead, move it to another day or time.

SET BOLD BOUNDARIES

It's one thing to schedule your habits in your calendar. It's quite another to make sure you actually have the time and freedom to do them at those times.

This one can be a bit tricky. This necessitates communicating them to your people and setting boundaries where necessary. In Chapter 16, "Shift #2: Rewire Limiting Beliefs," we mentioned the importance of setting boundaries (and how people pleasers struggle with this). I'll provide a quick summary here.

Setting Boundaries can require you to say "no" to those who depend on you, such as family, clients, or co-workers. These conversations are not always easy due to our human need for acceptance. Limiting self-beliefs that make us try to win acceptance through people pleasing or being nice can cause us to overcompensate by saying "yes" all the time, and to not say "no" enough of the time, which can lead to overwhelm and not having enough time for our body transformation habits.

So, we have to courageously (and tactfully) speak up and tell folks what we need. This may mean saying "no" to your manager about working late all the time or to not always jump when a family member makes a request. These conversations are delicate but necessary. If you struggle with saying "no," re-read the section on setting bolder boundaries in Chapter 16. There is also a boundary-setting exercise coming up in the Efficient Habits Implementation Plan. Review these items before having your next boundary-setting conversation. (It will be like having me in your ear, coaching you through it!)

THE EFFICIENT HABITS IMPLEMENTATION PLAN

GUIDELINES:

- Time Required: 10–15 minutes

- What You Will Need: Your digital calendar; a pen and something to write on
- Completing this plan will be fairly light and easy.

STEPS:

- ☐ Review the "Top-5 High Value Habits"
- ☐ Schedule your high value habits as anchors in your calendar
- ☐ Have successful boundary conversations

STEP #1: REVIEW THE "TOP-5 HIGH VALUE HABITS"

Again, they are:

1. Get religious about meal prep (1.5 hours per week if you batch cook).
2. Strength train often (2.25 hours per week—upper body (45 min), lower body (45 min), full body (45 min).
3. Stay connected to your why daily (1 hour per week; 10–15 min daily empowerment routine).
4. Take imperfect actions when you can't train formally.
5. Set anchors & boundaries (0.25 hour per week; just once per week).

As you can see, the total amount of time spent on these habits is roughly 3–5 hours per week if you're intentional. The key is to do them regularly. That's where scheduling comes into play.

STEP #2: SCHEDULE YOUR HIGH VALUE HABITS AS ANCHORS IN YOUR CALENDAR

Let's schedule these habits into your calendar in a very literal way.

You will use the concept of anchors that we covered in this chapter to set recurring time blocks to get your high value habits done each week.

To give you a head start, I've included an example of how to schedule these habits into your calendar on the next page.

Feel free to modify the days and durations of the anchor times you see in the example to make it work for you. For example, if you prefer to work out in the evenings versus the morning, shift the workout time anchors to the evenings.

I recommend that you schedule all five of the high value habits in your calendar (except for taking imperfect actions because that you'll do on the fly). Just review the imperfect actions you came up with in the Motivation Activation Plan in Chapter 17 and keep them in mind for those times when work or life keep you too busy to train or eat in an optimal way.

If you'd like to schedule additional habits beyond these Top 5 High Value Habits into your calendar, feel free to set anchors for as many as you'd like.

As you can see, there's still A LOT of empty space on your calendar to fit your life into it, while still getting your health habits done.

Make these habits part of your new lifestyle. They will start to become habits that you just do every week in and week out. As my clients all discover, with just a little bit of

Monday	Tuesday	Wednesday	Thursday
6:00 AM Daily Empowerment Routine (10–15 min)			
7:00 AM Upper Body WO (45 min)	**7:00 AM** Cardio (20–30 min)	**7:00 AM** Lower Body WO (45 min)	

planning, scheduling, and practice, balancing your life with your mind and body transformation goals can become practically painless and requires very little time!

STEP #3: HAVE SUCCESSFUL BOUNDARY CONVERSATIONS

Let's come up with a quick script for having a successful boundary conversation with the person who pulls at your time the most. The exercise will prepare you for the conversation in a way that eases your concerns about having this talk with them. Go through and answer the questions below:

A. Why is being your fittest and best important to you? You thought through this when you came up with your InPowerment Word with the Motivation Activa-

Friday	Saturday	Sunday
6:00 AM Daily Empowerment Routine (10–15 min)		
7:00 AM Full Body WO (45 min)	**7:00 AM** Cardio (0–30 min)	**7:00 AM** Cardio (20–30 min)
		7:00 PM Meal Prep (90 min)
		9:00 PM Plan Your Week/Anchors & Boundaries (15 min)

tion Plan in Chapter 17. Write it down again to make it present for yourself.

B. Do you feel that if you were to achieve this version of yourself that would make you a better or worse version of you for the people in your life? Would it make you a better coworker, spouse, or parent? Write down which one applies to this relationship.

C. What is a clear "ask" that you have for this person in your life that you need to set a boundary with? Be very specific about the amount of time or the specific time block you're going to say you're not available. For example, "I will no longer be available to stay late on Tuesday nights because I would like to start attending a fitness class at 6pm," or "I need to come in later on Thursday mornings because I want to start being more consistent with my morning workouts."

Now, combine A, B, and C to get your boundary conversation script.

It will read something like this:

"It's important for me to be my fittest and best because it helps me with my energy and I feel better overall. By having more energy and feeling better, I can be more productive and be the best contributor I can be for you. I'm asking for some extra time to come in later on Thursday mornings because I need that time each week to do Deekron's butt-kicking full body workout."

As you can see, using this template helps explain to the other person why you need the time, while also showing what's in it for them—a better version of you that will be contributing to them, better, and for longer.

Amazing work! You just fully completed this chapter.

Keep going and keep your transformation moving forward!

DON'T BELIEVE YOU DON'T HAVE TIME

We don't want to wait for the perfect time to do our habits. We also don't want to pretend that we don't have time to do them.

Remember that when the mind sees enough evidence of something, it will draw a conclusion and form a belief. If you have lots of things pulling at you and you struggle to find time for your transformation habits, it will start believing that you have no time. The more you say things like "I have no time" or "My life is too crazy," you reinforce the belief and this kills off any possibility of it being otherwise.

To not let limiting beliefs around time (or anything else for that matter) stop you, always reframe the conclusion as a question. Go from "I have no time" to "How can I find the time?"

The notion of not having time is not real. In fact, time itself isn't real. The concept of measuring time wasn't started till around 1,500 B.C. when the ancient Egyptians created the sundial. It's not clear how time was measured before that, other than to surmise that people tracked the movement of the sun and planned their days according to it.

Time is a made up construct and you can gain power over it by better understanding your relationship to it. Not finding time to do your transformation habits really comes down to the fact your approach is missing some of the elements we talk about in this book. Struggling to find time is usually a function of things like:

- Not saying "no" enough, lacking boundaries, or not asking for help.
- Overcompensating for subconscious unworthiness by chasing more accolades, money, status, or possessions.
- Overcompensating for subconscious unworthiness by trying to do everything perfectly which sucks up all your time.
- Lacking connection to why being your healthiest and best matters to you and your loved ones.
- Being distracted and triggered by outside influences that throw off your mood and tank your motivation.

Ultimately, the mistakes above will keep us thinking we don't have time. Additionally, if we spend our time on low-level activities which don't produce results, it might make us think that it's necessary to spend a ton of time just to make any kind of progress. This can also cause us to buy into the limiting belief of "I have no time."

Conversely, when you integrate the elements of the Efficient Habits Implementation Plan into your life, you'll realize that it doesn't take much time to get your habits done consistently, and you'll be motivated and grounded enough to find the time you need to maintain your body and health where you want them.

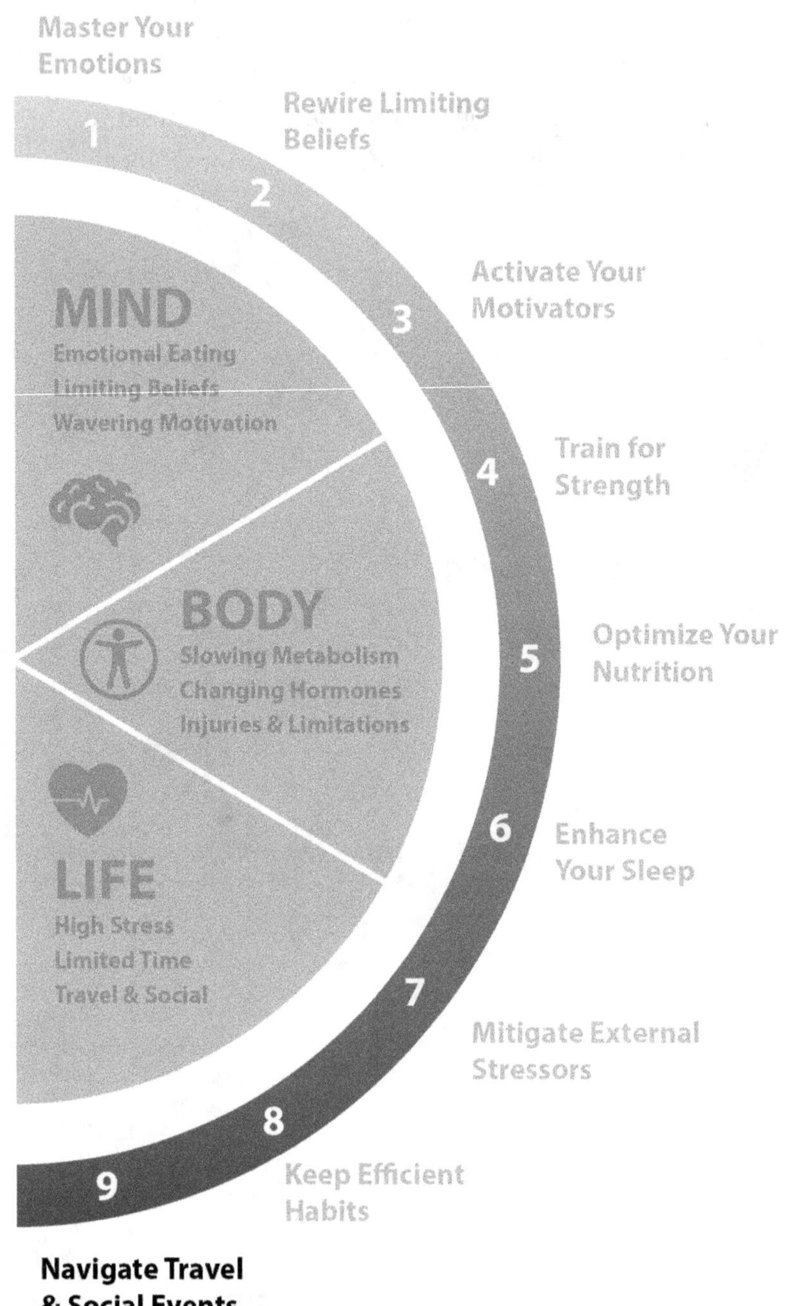

**Navigate Travel
& Social Events**

CHAPTER 25

SHIFT #9: Navigate Travel & Social Events

"Preparation for life is so important. Luck is what happens when preparedness meets opportunity. Opportunity is all around us. Are you prepared?"
—Earl Nightingale

Napoleon is quoted as having said, "A leader has a right to fail, but he (or she) does not have the right to be unprepared."

In order to keep our momentum up and not let commitments like travel or social events knock us off of our routine, we must be prepared with strategies for navigating them. Because, lord knows, they can be full of landmines for our habits and our waistline.

Most people rarely think ahead when it comes to the curveballs they'll face when they're on a trip or getting together with friends and family. Because these situations make it more likely to have rich food and drinks and skip our workouts, we have to account for them to avoid setbacks in our body and our health. In order get this step right, here is the key shift you will make:

KEY SHIFT

Go from being thrown off of your routine when traveling or attending social events, to preparing and having a plan for navigating these situations so you can enjoy them without getting set back.

This ninth and final shift will ensure you sustain your momentum even when you're away from home—on trips or at events. You will learn how to do this by going through this chapter and completing the Travel & Social Navigation Plan that's coming up soon.

THE APPROACH

The goal of this shift is to avoid the mistakes most people make when traveling or attending social events. Namely, they go in unprepared, without a strategy, and they get caught up in the moment.

Starting now, you're going to take a different approach that will have you better prepared and prevent these situations from killing your progress. The plan features flexibility and adapts to the different situations in which you might find yourself, including business trips, client dinners, happy hours with friends, family gatherings, etc.

Executing the steps in the Travel & Social Navigation Plan will help change your relationship with travel and social events from one where they throw you off your routine and negatively impact your health, to one where you are ready to handle them like a pro. Here are some key points to keep in mind.

PREPARING FOR TRIPS

To avoid the lousy food at airports, gas stations, and expo halls, you will make taking healthy snacks and supplements a part of your packing routine. You will also plan ahead to be more in control of when you will eat and how you will get some exercise during your trip. Here's how.

Packing Smart with the "Stay Optimal Travel Kit"

My first day at Accenture, as a young, newly-minted MBA about to jump into the waters of a management consulting career back in October of 1999 (jeez, time flies!), I remember sitting in orientation and being given some sage advice by the orientation leader. She said, because we were going to be traveling a lot (about 70–80% of the time), she recommended that we always have a second set of toiletries in our travel bag so we don't have to pack and unpack our toiletries all the time. This strategy made it easier to be prepared for our trips.

This concept can also be applied to our goal of being prepared for trips from a body transformation standpoint. One thing I teach my clients is to pack what I call a "Stay Optimal Travel Kit." This is a satchel or small bag you keep pre-packed and always-replenished so you can take it with you when you travel. You want it to include:

- Healthy snacks such as raw nuts, high-quality jerky, and healthy carbs like rice cakes or gluten-free granola bars.

- Supplements such as protein powder (along with your shaker cup), greens powder, fish oil pills, multivitamin, probiotics, and melatonin.
- A sleep satchel with an eye mask and ear plugs.
- An app or access to streaming workouts you can do virtually.
- A set of high-quality, adjustable resistance bands you can use if your hotel does not have a proper gym.

This travel kit will be invaluable in helping you maintain at least a minimum level of nutrition, exercise, and sleep that's in-line with your ongoing routine when you're at home.

Planning Ahead: Eating

If you know for sure you will be attending client lunches or dinners or having conference type meals during a work trip, it's best to assume that they will not be the healthiest options. The snacks in your Stay Optimal Travel Kit will help you get your macronutrients in if you're running around all day or pass on the food being offered.

On those days you know you will have a big dinner, you may want to do a longer fast that morning, and the following one, to create more budget for the calories you will be consuming at that dinner event.

Planning Ahead: Exercising

Before going on a trip, it makes sense to plan ahead to see what facilities you'll have access to. This will enable you to stay in your regular workout groove, especially when it comes to getting in your strength training.

If you know your facilities will be limited, you can pack some light equipment, like a set of resistance bands, a jump rope, or a thin yoga mat, to help you stay active. If going by car, you can even throw some equipment, like some adjustable dumbbells, in the trunk.

ACING YOUR SOCIAL EVENTS

Here are some go-to strategies to keep in your back pocket. They will prevent overdoing it with food or drinking in social situations and ensure you navigate these events with poise.

Booze Control

In Chapter 12, "Challenge #9: Travel & Social," you learned about my "Half-Tank" strategy, which advises that you eat a little something healthy before heading out to an event. This ensures you don't show up famished and prevents overeating. It also provides a bit of food to absorb alcohol if you start the event with drinks.

Another strategy I teach for navigating social events is what I call , "The Preset Liquor Limit." It works like this: before you get to an event, you will proactively set a realistic limit of drinks for yourself. Keep this number in mind and make a promise around it to yourself or, ideally, to someone who can hold you to it. This can prevent having "a few too many."

Pair Big Events with Big Workouts

I came up with this strategy years ago to help me survive big Thanksgiving feasts. The idea is to boost your metabolism right before going to a big-eating event so you can have more of a buffer to absorb the extra food and calories you'll be having.

Do an intense strength training workout, ideally lower body since that's the most taxing on the metabolism, as close as possible to the event. Basically, workout, shower, get ready, and head out.

Remember, an intense strength training workout (or HIIT cardio workout) creates the afterburn effect, which elevates your metabolism for many hours after your workout is over. It also taps into your glycogen stores (in your muscles and liver). This means your body burns through the glycogen from the carbs you ate previously and is now depleted.

Any new carbs you eat get funneled to your depleted muscles stores **first**. This means there is a much lower chance that they'll get deposited into your fat cells. Muscles get first priority, and since they're depleted, they will suck up any carbs you eat like a sponge.

That means the bread stuffing, potatoes, and pecan pie I have at Thanksgiving won't affect my waistline very much.

By the way, this strategy is not limited to Thanksgiving only. You can use it any time, including weddings, client dinners, birthday parties, and the like to give yourself more cushion and more freedom to indulge without the guilt or impact on your waist.

Just keep in mind that you have to earn this privilege by working out intensely enough before the event. Taking your dog for a walk isn't going to cut it. (Sorry, Rover).

MAKING THE RIGHT CHOICE

This mindset strategy creates clarity when faced with a "should I or shouldn't I" decision. For example, when wondering if you should have another slice of that scrumptious pizza or debating with yourself whether you should skip a happy hour or go to it.

Here's how it helped my client Eric, the former airline executive who worked with us to achieve a six-pack at 65.

Eric is very social and regularly attends Saturday night get-togethers, which usually involve plenty of food and drink. With rich foods, desserts, and alcohol flowing, Eric would often find it difficult to strike the right balance in these situations.

While he wanted to respect the group's norms and eat the foods being provided, he also did not want to not splurge too much and wipe out the progress he had made during the week with his body transformation progress.

So what's the solution?

Simple.

View it through the lens of happiness.

When torn between indulging versus depriving, use this question as your filter: "Which choice would make me feel the happiest?"

For instance, ask: Will it make me the happiest to have this drink, toasting this person and getting to relax? Or will having this drink make me feel bad and stressed out? Ask yourself these questions and feel into them. Your gut won't lead you wrong. (No pun intended!)

This practice can act as the filter you need to make the right choice next time you're faced with a tough decision around food in a social setting, or otherwise.

So there you have it, strategies to prevent trips and social events from setting you back, and how to make the right decision even when you're torn. Feel free to modify or add more go-to strategies that can allow you to take better control of eating and drinking at social events to make it work for you.

Next, let's put these strategies into action.

THE TRAVEL & SOCIAL NAVIGATION PLAN

GUIDELINES:

- Time Required: 5–10 minutes
- What You Will Need: Basic details about your upcoming trip or social event

STEPS:

- ☐ Pack smart and plan ahead for trips
- ☐ Plan your travel strategy
- ☐ Plan your social strategy

Now, dive in, go through the steps below, and make this shift!

STEP #1: CREATE YOUR "STAY OPTIMAL TRAVEL KIT"

Before you travel, you will pack healthy snacks, supplements, light workout equipment, and other simple tools to take in your luggage or vehicle.

Write out some items that you can take with you for each category below. Feel free to use the example items provided and to add/subtract as needed:

- healthy snacks (mixed nuts, rice cakes or crackers, healthy jerky)
- supplements (protein powder, fish oil pills, multi-vitamins, greens powder)
- sleep satchel (eye mask, ear plugs, app with white noise or sleep sounds)
- streaming workouts via an app you can do virtually (YouTube playlist, Instagram playlist)
- light workout equipment (a set of resistance bands, ab roller, small hand weights, ankle weights)

Pro Tip: Amazon has most of what you'll need to put in your Stay Optimal Travel Kit but feel free to shop locally as well.

Now, schedule a small time slot in your calendar to block off time to buy or secure these items. Make sure you put your Stay Optimal Travel Kit in your usual luggage or in your vehicle and be sure to REPLENISH any items that run out when you get back from your trip or your workday. You can also use your weekly meal prep anchor time to replenish your kit.

STEP #2: PLAN YOUR TRAVEL STRATEGY

Think through each one of the areas below so you can be ready for anything that your trip may throw at you.

Think About What and When You'll Eat

Think about the dynamics of your trip and how it will affect food choices and eating times. Will your days be full of running around or a lot of sitting around? Will you have time and appetite to eat when you wake up or will you be eating big meals at night due to client dinners? Will there be healthy food options you can choose from or will you be surrounded by poor choices and fast food restaurants? Will you fast while you're in transit or during your trip as a strategy to control calories? If you have house calls and can not eat during these times, will you have to stop and eat, even if it's in your car, before heading into a house for an appointment?

Write out some thoughts for what your situation will be like and how you will manage your nutrition, including consuming your packed snacks to get through your days.

Think About How and When You'll Exercise

It is recommended to get the minimum effective dose of physical activity, even while traveling. This will keep your motivation and momentum going.

Think through what your schedule will be like (i.e., how busy) and decide ahead of time if you will get minimal exercise (e.g., just walking or imperfect actions), light exercise (e.g., doing some shorter workouts in your hotel), or full on exercise (e.g., finding a local gym near your hotel). There's no right or wrong answer, just look to balance continuing your progress versus practicality.

STEP #3: PLAN YOUR SOCIAL STRATEGY

Let's think through how we will implement the strategies we learned to help navigate social events without letting them hurt our waistline or our momentum.

Apply the half-tank strategy and come up with a go-to snack that is light, healthy, and practical (no cooking required) that will fill you up partially before heading out to your event. Examples include some hummus with carrot sticks, a serving of yogurt with nuts, some oatmeal with fruit, or a small can or pouch of tuna with rice cakes.

Use the preset liquor limit before your event, and stick to it. What do you feel is a good number of drinks to which you'd like to limit yourself? What is a mental note you can make to remind yourself of this limit before you enter the event? And if you are going with someone else to the event would you feel comfortable asking them to keep you accountable to your limit?

Remember to use situational happiness so you're making the right choices. Ask yourself what will make you the happiest—having that extra serving of food (or drink), or keeping to your health habits?

OK, now wait a minute . . .

Are you seriously going to tell me that you just completed the ninth and final shift chapter?

What!

Amazing work!

You're so close now to your new future, you can taste it!

Just two chapters to go.

Don't quit on me now, buster.

You've got this!

PART IV

Your Future

CHAPTER 26

Add Support for Success

"You cannot solve a problem with the same mind that created it."
—Albert Einstein

When Tracy finished her six-month program with my team and I at the InPowerment Company, we had a final call to celebrate her success. She had lost nearly twenty pounds and was stable at her desired weight, even allowing for a piece of cake or glass of wine whenever she felt like it. But the best part was how she ***felt***.

"I feel completely different in how I look. I feel really confident. I have an element of respect for myself that is carrying over into the rest of my life."

She smiled at me, her whole face radiant. "I just feel so much more in control, and I have all the tools I need now. It just feels so sustainable."

I smiled with her, happy to see her so changed from the embarrassed, frustrated, and scared woman she had been just a few months ago.

She kept going, "And you know what? The guilt is completely gonc. You know, where you have a piece of chocolate and then spend the next day starving yourself to make up for it? Or you have a couple of glasses of wine and feel so guilty you go off alcohol for a month? That massive oscillation between ***all in and all out is completely gone.***"

She paused, smiled again and said, "That's just such a relief, it really is!"

I asked her how she felt about continuing the mind, body and life transformation habits we had taught her.

She said, "I have a level of knowledge that I never had before, about training and nutrition and sleep and emotional well being. I just didn't have the tools before. It's so ingrained now, I don't even need to think about it. I think this is probably the best investment I've ever made in myself."

"Thank you," I said, "that is why I do what I do. I'm so happy for you."

"But Deekron," she said, "you know what the most valuable part was? It was all of our conversations, especially around mindset. You continuously brought me back to why I'm doing this, why it matters to me. That shifted everything for me."

So, you made it through all nine shifts! Excellent work hanging in there!

You've seen, first-hand, that it takes more than just diet and exercise to achieve lasting change in your body after forty. Which is why *The Nine Shifts* method addresses all of the main challenges of mind, body and life, from the inside out.

Ideally, coming this far has inspired you to take action. To stop waiting and to start reaching, anew, for the body, health, and life you've been waiting for.

The good news is that you now have the playbook to achieve your desired body and health, and keep it for good.

But you're pretty smart and you know that it takes more than just reading a book to get the results we're after. It's about executing what we've learned. Implementing new habits and adopting a new lifestyle that supports our new body. As you know now, the mind—with its comfort zone, and old, ingrained patterns—will resist change and try to keep us stuck.

Getting over this inertia—with an aging body and a packed schedule—takes a lot. That's why it's so hard to get back on track when we lose momentum. If you struggled with this in the past, then you're already wired to struggle again. (Sorry, but that's just the reality of it.)

Luckily, studies have shown that if we take the really wise step of getting the right support around us, it greatly improves our chances of success. Now, I'm not saying this only because I want to win your business and have my team and I at the InPowerment Company support you in your transformation. If I'm being honest, we do. But, more than that, I don't want you to have to struggle like I did for 30+ years.

I didn't make my greatest progress until I started getting professional help with this, in all the different domains. The nutrition bit alone is hard enough. If your mindset, old habits or outside obstacles have been stopping you, like they do with most people, it will be very difficult to solve on one's own.

This is where getting support becomes invaluable.

Getting different minds around you, that don't have the same patterns and fears as you, empowers you to shift out of your usual ways of thinking and operating. If those minds have already experienced success in transforming their body, then that's even better. If those minds are skilled in helping people who face the same obstacles as you to achieve your desired result—in a way that actually lasts—then that's the best option of all.

By reading this far you've learned about what it takes to transform your body permanently by implementing *The Nine Shifts* into your life. You have the knowledge you need to reach your goals.

The only thing you have to do from here is to choose whether you go it alone or get support.

As you're deciding, remember these three things:

1. Transforming your body permanently isn't easy.
2. Getting quality support saves you time, frustration, and improves your chances of lasting success.
3. Get the best help you can afford.

Here's a bit more about these three considerations.

1. TRANSFORMING YOUR BODY PERMANENTLY ISN'T EASY

As you've seen, true, lasting change happens at the level of the subconscious mind and our emotions. Only by gaining awareness of how we're wired can we overcome the mental obstacles that drive up stress, cause us to eat or drink emotionally, keep us stuck in our comfort zone or in overcompensation, and have our motivation slip.

Because most approaches don't start with the mind, the long-term failure rate is high. Even more so if you've struggled with your body in the past. Like I said, I believe that this is one reason why 70% of the U.S. is overweight or obese.

Sure, there might be a few folks out there who can figure this out on their own without doing a program or getting support. But don't let the #transformationtuesday posts fool you. It's usually a very small percentage of folks who most likely don't have your metabolism, limitations, or responsibilities.

2. GETTING QUALITY SUPPORT SAVES YOU TIME, FRUSTRATION AND MONEY

Having the right support around you will save you time. First, by helping you avoid hours upon hours of reading, researching, and experimenting. Granted, reading this book has brought you a long way in gaining knowledge and proven strategies. But, like with anything else, once you get going you will inevitably have questions, and that will take knowledge that you still don't have.

Second, it saves you time-to-results. Doing it on your own can keep you stuck, trying and experimenting, for years or even decades (like in my case). But when someone can take you by the hand and lead you straight to your goal, you save a lot of time. I didn't see my best results until I started working with the right coaches.

This also helps you save frustration. As you know, the mind hates it when we fail. The more we fail at something the less likely we are to keep trying. However, with the right guidance you can avoid feeling this way. Even if you do have a bad week or two, the right support will help you shift out of frustration and keep you taking action. But left to our own devices, that frustration can trigger your limiting beliefs:"I just can't seem to figure this out" or "Maybe I was just meant to be fat," or "I just don't have the time for this right now." This, in turn, kills our motivation and knocks us out of action until we get frustrated by our inaction to the point where we feel desperate enough to force ourselves to try again.

Third, investing in the right support to get to your goal efficiently, with minimal friction and hassle, ends up saving you a lot of money over the long run. This is true from the aspect of not having to keep investing in some new thing every year, like fancy cardio equipment, a boot camp, useless pills and supplements, detoxes, going back to (another) personal trainer, etc. It's also true from the standpoint of avoiding health-related issues in the future. If we don't get this right and go into our later years overweight and unhealthy, we have to start spending money on doctor's visits, medication, treatments, possible operations, or potential catastrophic events like heart attacks or strokes.

And of course, time is money, so there's that, too.

3. GET THE BEST HELP YOU CAN AFFORD

Obviously, getting support comes down to your willingness and availability to invest. Your chances of success are much better with the proper guidance—getting the right mentor or coach is essential. This is why every great athlete and high performing CEO has one. Some have several. Top athletes like Tom Brady and Lebron James spend more than $1 million per year on their bodies.

PAY LESS NOW OR PAY MORE LATER

There used to be a TV commercial that was running in the 1980's for FRAM Oil Filter showing two mechanics working in a garage. The first mechanic is the one speaking to the camera, while his coworker Joe is rebuilding an engine behind him. The first mechanic advises us to buy the right oil filter so we don't have bigger issues that can require a full engine rebuild later on. A full engine rebuild with Joe in the back room costs a lot more than buying a good oil filter. "You can pay me now, or you can pay him (Joe) later," the first mechanic advises.

It's the same with your health. You can make a smaller investment with the right program now, or you can pay your doctor a lot more later. Hiring the right support to get you to your goal now saves you more money in the long run. Not to mention gives you a much better quality of life.

Now, you may not have a million dollars per year to spend on your body. Fortunately, you don't need to spend that much. But do your best to invest as much as you can. Oftentimes, when I speak to folks who really need support to turn their health around and are suffering, they get stopped due to finances. Obviously, finances need to be considered; I get it. At the same time, many people develop a knee-jerk reaction to investing in something, even if it's for themselves, and default to "I can't afford it" without even thinking it through.

A better response is to ask "How can I afford it?" This was the lesson from the bestselling book by Robert Kiyosaki, *Rich Dad, Poor Dad.*[72] With some creativity and enough desire—by being present to our why and future pain that might be coming—we can usually find a way.

One of my mentors would even say "If someone wants to work with you badly enough, they'll even drive Uber on the weekends." (He's not wrong.)

A one-time, permanent solution to your health saves time, money, and frustration and is not a luxury. Thus, we owe it to ourselves to stretch ourselves and get the best help we can afford. Yes, we need to take a leap of faith but taking that leap helps you break free of the mind's limitations and comfort zone. That, in itself, is ***priceless.***

THE NINE SHIFTS TRANSFORMS MORE THAN JUST YOUR BODY

When my clients start to transform via *The Nine Shifts* mind-first method, some neat things start to happen. Of course, they start shedding body fat, building muscle tone, and improving their health overall. Moreover, they start taking more risks and give themselves more freedom to fail. They put less pressure on themselves, and those around them, to have to be perfect all the time. They think and perform better and enter into more of a flow. They start prioritizing themselves and setting the boundaries they need to get their body transformation and self-care habits done consistently.

Not only do they gain greater compassion for themselves, but for others too.

They start to realize that we all have limiting beliefs and they can really make us struggle, be unhappy, and overcompensate. In my opinion, this is the ultimate ROI—no longer having to overcompensate. Allowing the real you to emerge and to impact those around you.

My clients have produced amazing outcomes as a result of their total transformation. Some have gained the confidence to go out and find a better, higher paying job. Others have mended contentious relationships at work.

And then there's Andy. About four months after completing our program, where he successfully lost weight and got a lot stronger, he lost his mother. Stricken with grief, he suffered a minor heart attack while he was at work. His doctor told him if he hadn't lost the weight and improved his health in time, he might not have survived that heart attack.

His family is eternally grateful for the work we did with him. We're truly touched by their sentiment and are so glad he survived to tell us about it. But really, for us it was just another day's work.

AN OPTION THAT SAVES YOU TIME

If you're like most executives, you value time over money. This means you're willing to make an investment in speed, knowledge, and predictable results. *The Nine Shifts* works, and it works every time that it's implemented correctly.

My team and I have worked with 120+, over-40 professionals and counting. We've gotten really good at customizing the action plans to each client's unique needs.

You can think of it like building a house.

This book is like your blueprint. You can go off and build a house (i.e., your body) with these instructions on your own.

Or my team and I can come in, and we'll build it together with you. This way, you can be sure that the foundation is solid and your house will not collapse on you in the middle of the night, the electricity is sound and a fire will not break out when you plug in your toaster, and your plumbing will not cause a flood and damage your expensive carpets.

One of my mentors would often say, "Information is not transformation." There's something to be said about having experts and mentors in your corner every step of the way, answering your questions, teaching you the right knowledge, guiding you to start new habits, and making you sure you learn how to integrate them into your life, for life.

Outsource the transformation of your body and your health to us. We'll ensure your success.

When you're ready. click on the QR code on this page to book a time to connect with me or someone on my team. We're happy to hear more about your situation and assess if we're the right fit to permanently get you to where you want to be.

CHAPTER 27

Your Time Is Now

"Go for it now. The future is promised to no one."
—Wayne Dyer

Part of my job as a coach and body transformation expert is to motivate and inspire people to take action.

Remember, the mind will resist action, push away from change, and come up with damn good reasons to keep us stuck in the familiar.

To this point, I've given you many tools to help you overcome the mind's resistance by connecting with your "why" and tapping into inspiration instead of willpower. I also pointed out that fear and pain avoidance can also be motivating. In fact, even moreso. When we get present to the potential of the pain that may result if we continue to procrastinate and stay stuck, it can override the comfort zone and get us into action. In a sense, we're scaring ourselves into action, but we're coming from a good place.

All this to say that creating urgency is our best friend when it comes to avoiding a future that's full of health issues, suffering, and a poor quality of life. In that spirit—and with your permission—I'd like to deliver a few pieces of hard truth in order to create some urgency and light a fire under your derriere. These are reality-check type reminders that I believe we, as people, need to hear more often . . .

TRUTH #1: THINGS ARE MORE COMPLICATED NOW

Keeping our body in a good place is easy in our twenties and thirties, but for most of us it gets harder once we cross over into our forties. Having read through the challenges in Part II of this book, you know now that being at our life stage and having our level of responsibility, poses unique challenges.

An aging body, a slowing metabolism, declining hormones, high stress levels, limiting beliefs, and not enough time create obstacles that make reaching our goal more difficult.

Years of high stress, medication, yo-yo dieting, undersleeping and poor eating habits can eventually catch up to us. The majority of my clients come to me with numerous complications that make it harder to lose weight. Complications such as high blood sugar levels, low testosterone, thyroid issues, mental health challenges, aches and pains, inflammation, high cholesterol. Not to mention, like most of us, they have to battle limited time, lack of motivation, and lots of responsibilities.

So yeah, this life stage makes things harder for sure.

All the more reason to get started now.

TRUTH #2: THE LONGER YOU WAIT THE HARDER IT GETS

This one is obvious but worth mentioning for the sake of creating urgency. The more we delay getting our body to a good place, the harder things get; until eventually the goal slips out of reach, it becomes too late, and we have to accept a fate that involves not liking what we see in pictures or not being able to wear our favorite clothes any longer. The more time that goes by, the more the metabolism slows, the more our hormones decline, the more injuries and limitations our body may face.

Another thing most people take for granted is that their situation will stay the same. But this is not always the case. A parent or child may fall sick and require a lot of our time and energy. We may deal with a major life stressor like divorce or death of a loved one. We may lose our job or have to move.

A lot can go wrong. We can't assume we'll have the same amount of time and stability we have now.

If such hardships come to pass, and you've already gotten your body to a good place (and know how to maintain it efficiently and consistently in the face of those hurdles), then you'll be ***really glad*** you handled it when you did. If not, you'll ***regret*** not having started sooner because now it will be much harder.

TRUTH #3: TOMORROW IS NOT GUARANTEED

Due to the mind's comfort zone, most humans don't make a change until something drastic happens. For some of us, it takes receiving a scary health report from the doctor. My client Tracy's wake up call came when her A1C had reached a prediabetic level. For others, change doesn't come until we realize how our behaviors are making our loved ones feel.

My client Nate is the CEO of a luxury home construction company. He was about sixty pounds overweight and, admittedly, didn't keep great health habits. Having steaks, subs, and drinks were a weekly, if not daily, occurrence. He had never stopped to think about making a change in earnest until one day his teenage-daughter confessed to him, in tears, that she secretly feared he wasn't going to be around for much longer. That conversation changed everything and spurred him into action.

For the unlucky ones and their families, change doesn't come until we're faced with the unexpected death of a friend or loved one. A great example is that of my friend Robert, who I met through the Armenian community while I was living in New York. He was the coach of our Armenian church's youth basketball team and a real pillar of our community. Successful at work, he was a senior executive at one of the nation's top recruiting firms. Less successful with his health, he had always been overweight.

One day he came home from a long day at the office and suffered a major heart attack, which ended his life. He left behind a wife, two kids, and shockwaves throughout our community. He was forty-five.

Yup, life can be harsh.

Know that I give these examples as a friendly-but-firm reminder.

If your body and health are not in a good place . . .

PLEASE DON'T WAIT

I took a long time to make a change.

The catalyst for me wasn't as drastic as some of the examples I gave above, fortunately. For me it was the pain of hitting a "rock bottom" point in my life when I got divorced. That finally pushed me over the edge and had me say "Enough is enough!"

The cost of me waiting as long as I did was that I robbed myself of being the best version of myself for many years. The consequences can be higher than this for many others. So please . . . don't wait until:

- You get a scary prognosis from your doctor.
- Your spouse starts losing interest.
- Your coworkers or managers start wondering if you still "got what it takes."
- You hate what you see in the mirror.
- You suffer a medical emergency.

Remember, your life can unexpectedly get even more complicated by a hardship that robs you of time to focus on you and your needs.

The time to take a committed step to become your best is always now.

This book has shown you the path.

I've given you the blueprint.

It's the same blueprint I wish I had in my teens, twenties and thirties.

Writing, and then having to totally re-write, this book was the hardest thing I've ever done (and I've done a lot of hard stuff!). But I wrote it so that you don't have to struggle for decades like I did. I wrote it so you can have a clear plan to end your struggles and achieve your desired body and health, and to—finally—keep it for good.

It's time for you to shift from learning to implementing.

It's time for you to shift your life and transform.

It's time for you to shift out of your struggles and permanently gain the confidence, health, and peace you've been craving.

Please don't wait.

CHOOSE YOUR FUTURE

Some good news. Six months after completing her coaching program with us, Tracy texted me a screenshot of her latest blood work test results and her A1C had returned to normal. Diabetes was officially off the table and was going to stay off as far as Tracy was concerned.

More than two years after she finished her coaching program with us, Tracy sent me an email with a picture of her and her husband skiing in the alps. They both looked so happy. Her new life had taken hold. More than two years after adopting *The Nine Shifts* transformation method, Tracy was still healthy, happy, and ***feeling great about her body and her future.*** (What an amazing turnaround from where she started!)

This could be your future, too.

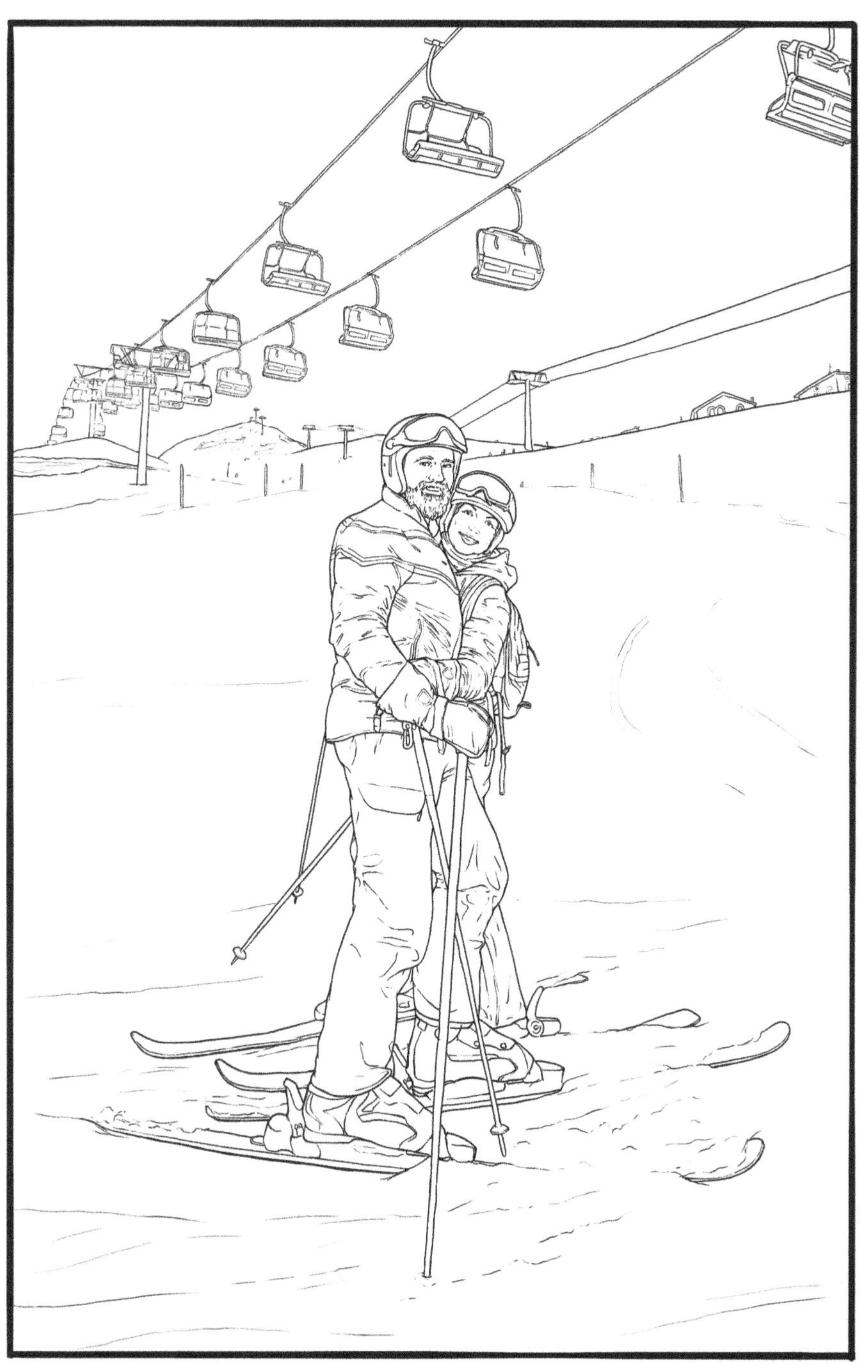

Next Steps

To continue your journey to permanent body transformation, feel free to take advantage of the resources below.

ACCESS YOUR BONUSES

You will find worksheets that support the action plans in each shift chapter as well as other resources for successfully implementing *The Nine Shifts* into your life, at this link: https://thenineshifts.com/downloads

LEARN HOW TO MEAL PREP PROPERLY

Optimizing your nutrition is one of the most important shifts to make to achieve the lasting body, health, and energy you seek. A key habit for making this shift is preparing your meals on a weekly basis. This allows you to take control of what you're eating and not have to rely on outside sources of food, which are not always optimal for our health and our goals.

Meal prepping the right way takes some practice. We want to make this an efficient, effortless process so that it doesn't require constantly having to decide what to eat, cook, and clean.

I do my meal prep in about 90 minutes on Sundays and never have to worry about cooking or cleaning during the week. Because this is such an important habit to adopt and skill to develop, I've put together a "behind-the-scenes" training video so you see exactly how I shop and cook my foods when I do my meal prep each week.

My exclusive training video will show you exactly how it's done. You can learn more and purchase it as this link below, or by scanning the QR code provided:

thenineshifts.com/meal-prep-training

AN OPTION FOR ACCELERATING YOUR TRANSFORMATION

From my experience coaching over-40 professionals, I know first-hand that you often have pretty complicated situations you're juggling. Between your career, family, and other life obligations, you have little time for much else. Adding another thing to your plate, especially something as daunting as change, which the mind naturally resists, might make you hesitant.

I get it.

As mentioned, to guide you in successfully implementing *The Nine Shifts*, I've assembled and trained a team of elite coaches to support you with your journey.

It goes without saying that results come the fastest when we have a well-qualified mentor that steers us clear of mistakes and keeps us on track. I've made the best progress in my body, career, and happiness when I've worked with experienced coaches and caring mentors.

If and when you feel ready, know that you have a resource in us for outsourcing your body transformation goals.

YOUR INVITATION

If you're ready to cut-to-the-chase and want to learn about how we support over-40 professionals to overcome their challenges and implement *The Nine Shifts* into their life—so you can look, feel and perform your best immediately—apply for a complimentary Breakthrough Call via this link: http://thenineshifts.com/call

Alternatively, you can scan the QR code below with your phone.

On this 15-minute phone call, we will learn more about your situation, share some insights, and determine if our In-Powered Body transformation program, featuring the *Nine Shifts*, is right for you. If it is, we will invite you to a longer Transformation Session. Neither of these calls carry a cost or obligation for readers of *The Nine Shifts*, so feel free to take advantage of this opportunity to gain greater clarity and explore our program more closely. We look forward to connecting with you.

Motion Traxx (If you'd like to check it out, here's the link. Or scan the QR code to download and get five free sessions when you sign up; no credit card required. **www.motiontraxx.com**

Acknowledgments

Naturally, I need to start with Mom and Dad, the greatest parents (and now, grandparents) that anyone can ever ask for. Love you both with all my heart and am beyond grateful for all you have instilled in Ara and me.

To my baby brother, Ara, for giving me the courage to break the rules, teaching me how important creativity can be, and for always inspiring so many of us with your incredible passion and musical talent. Being part of the fabric of the House and Techno scene in NYC alongside you for all those years were some of the best days (and nights) of my life, all thanks to you. ("Stay Young. Love Techno." . . . forever.)

To my niece Violet: For blessing us with your constant joy, endless curiosity, and delightful storytelling. I can't wait till you read this book! (And to Becka for always making sure she's always well taken care of!)

To Dr. Z., my brother from another mother. Thank you for always looking out for me, teaching me about medicine and science, peer reviewing the science in this book, and being a best friend and great sidekick during so many fun nights out together. Shukran.

To Nick P., thank you for your empathy and undying support, mon pote. Je suis très reconnaissant.

To the rest of my Miami squad: Mando, DLaw, Verde, Eddie and Dude Bro. We're the poster boys of staying young at heart. Let's keep it up, fellas!

To my favorite bosses: Scott Stansfield, my first ever real boss, mentor, and friend to this day. To Clarence Mitchell, the coolest partner I ever worked for and someone who I am privileged to consider my dear friend. To Sevag, a brother and friend who always made me feel valued for my contributions while pushing me to stretch and grow and learn what it really takes to run a successful business.

To my Michigan squad: Hash, Manny V, Rob, Gerry, Aureliano, and the rest of you guys and gals. Go Blue!

To all those who toiled alongside me to make this book possible: Angela and Patrick, my amazing editors who were incredibly undaunted by the complexity of this project, while being the best sounding board and honest guides I could've ever hoped for. To Adameus (aka "The Other Adam Levine"), my incredible art director and designer (and friend and brother and fellow suffering Knicks fan) since 2009, thanks to your amazing strategic mind and capable hands, this book can express itself beautifully to the human eye.

To my soul sisters, Manu and Drea. For always holding space for me and providing the strong, nurturing, wisdom

I need to hear. Not to mention your support in PR, marketing, and branding help that I have no doubt will help put this book over the top.

To my favorite coaches: Ted Santos, if you ever read this please know that I'll never forget all of the powerful transformation lessons you instilled in me. Matt Tracy (IFBB Pro), a true gentleman and a gentle giant who stepped in to help me during my darkest weeks of contest prep. Thanks for helping me pull through, big guy. To Neil Talbot, your empathetic and loving coaching always makes me beam with optimism and confidence. Thank you, good sir.

To my best training partner and spotter of all time, Armen Caprielian. Thanks for sharing this passion with me since we were teens. So glad we're still at it!

To my cousin Karine, who didn't give up on me when I was stubborn and stood by me until I was ready to be introduced to the beautiful world of transformation.

To the 1.5 million Armenians who were slaughtered during the Armenian Genocide of 1915 in Ottoman Turkey, we will never forget.

To Tony Robbins, Landmark Education, and all of the other courses, programs, and content creators that have helped me elevate my mind and body.

To Rebeca my girlfriend: Thank you for being the spice that brings me alive. What we have is so special. No pensé que una mujer como tu existe. No pensé que un amor como nuestro sera posible. Gracias por estar en mi vida, muñeca.

To all the others who contributed to this project: my photographer Chris Williams, my marketing consultant Katie Anderson, and my VA Jessica Aguirre. Thank you, guys!

To Stephen D., for coaching our clients with such great care and attention to detail, your commitment and support give me the freedom to run.

To all the bands that fuel my workouts, especially Godsmack, Disturbed, Chevelle, The Peppers, Metallica, Sabbath, Priest, Dio (RIP) and Maiden: keep rockin' fellas.

To all my clients who invested in my program, partnered with my team and I, and trusted us to take them on a journey to better their lives. This book would not be possible without you.

Finally, to anyone else who rooted for me, supported me, taught me, partnered with me, loved me, trusted me, or stood for me throughout the years: thank you! Know that I will do my very best to pay forward all that you've ever done for me.

About the Author

Dikran "Deekron" Krikorian is zealous about personal growth and living true to one's passions. Always believing in "walking the talk," he left behind a prestigious corporate career as a strategy consultant to empower people to achieve their best self.

Deekron earned an MBA from the Ross School of Business at The University of Michigan. He holds certifications in Functional Nutrition & Metabolism (FNMS by Sam Miller Science) as well as Pain Free Performance Specialist (PPSC by Dr. John Rusin). He's done deep immersive transformation work, training live with experts such as Tony Robbins, Les Brown, and Bob Proctor. He's also worked directly with elite mindset and body transformation coaches.

Deekron is the founder of the award-winning fitness app, Motion Traxx, which was featured for over a year by Apple in The App Store.

He competed in a natural bodybuilding competition at the age of 50 (placing second) and ran the New York City Marathon in 2011, a day before his 40th birthday. His favorite sport is skiing; he was a part-time ski instructor and ski racer, earning silver in a coalition cup and on the NASTAR Alpine Racing circuit as a teenager.

He was born in Romania (to an Armenian dad and Romanian mom) grew up in Queens (the most ethnically diverse neighborhood on the planet) and currently lives in Miami, Florida, his happy place.

Notes

CHAPTER 1

1 "Overweight & Obesity Statistics," U.S. Department of Health and Human Services, https://www.niddk.nih.gov/health-information/health-statistics/overweight-obesity

2 Joni Sweet, "Think You're Metabolically Healthy? Only 12% of Americans Fit the Bill," Healthline, December 6, 2018, https://www.healthline.com/health-news/what-does-it-mean-to-be-metabolically-healthy

3 "Obesity: Symptoms, Causes, Treatment", WebMD, June 28, 2023, https://www.webmd.com/obesity/what-obesity-is

4 US Department of Health and Human Services. Centers for Disease Control., "National Diabetes Statistics Report: Estimates of Diabetes and Its Burden in the United States," Centers for Disease Control, 2020, https://www.cdc.gov/diabetes/pdfs/data/statistics/national-diabetes-statistics-report.pdf

5 "Overweight and Obesity Fact Sheet: Health Consequences," n.d., http://www.wvdhhr.org/bph/oehp/hp/obesity/fact_consequences.htm

6 "Fast Food Restaurants in the US - Number of Businesses", IBIS World, October 17, 2023, https://www.ibisworld.com/industry-statistics/number-of-businesses/fast-food-restaurants-united-states/ and Colman Andrews, "States With the Most (and Fewest) Fast Food Restaurants Per Person", 247WallSt, November 27, 20222, https://247wallst.com/special-report/2022/11/27/states-with-the-most-and-fewest-fast-food-restaurants-per-capita/

7 Michelle Harven, "How ultra-processed food has changed our minds, bodies, and culture", June 27, 2023, https://the1a.org/segments/how-ultra-processed-food-has-integrated-into-our-minds-bodies-and-culture/

8 "America's Eating Habits: Changes and Consequences", U.S. Department of Agriculture, Economic Research Service, Food and Rural Economics Division. Agriculture Information Bulletin No. 750, Anthony

E. Gallo, “Chapter 9: Food Advertising in the United States”, USDA, AIB 750 , USDA/VERS 179, https://www.ers.usda.gov/webdocs/publications/42215/5838_aib750i_1_.pdf

9 Marschall S. Runge, MD, PhD, “Weighing the Facts: The Tough Truth About Weight Loss”, Michigan Medicine, April 12, 2017, https://www.michiganmedicine.org/health-lab/weighing-facts-tough-truth-about-weight-loss, and Marcel Schwantes, *Inc.*, July 26, 2016, https://www.inc.com/marcel-schwantes/science-says-92-percent-of-people-dont-achieve-goals-heres-how-the-other-8-perce.html

CHAPTER 2

10 Jennifer Kunst Ph.D., “There's Only One Way to Change: Slowly, Over Time: You've Got to Take It One Step at a Time,” Psychologytoday.com, September 21, 2011, https://www.psychologytoday.com/us/blog/headshrinkers-guide-the-galaxy/201109/theres-only-one-way-change-slowly-over-time

CHAPTER 3

11 James Loehr, Jim Loehr, and Tony Schwartz, *The Power of Full Engagement: Managing Energy, Not Time, Is the Key to High Performance and Personal Renewal* (Amsterdam, Netherlands: Amsterdam University Press, 2005).

CHAPTER 4

12 “Stress and Eating”, *American Psychological Association*, 2013, https://www.apa.org/news/press/releases/stress/2013/eating

13 Arthur Lefford, "The Influence of Emotional Subject Matter on Logical Reading," *Journal of General Psychology* 34: 127–151.

14 “You are your Brain”, Cleveland Clinic, https://healthybrains.org/brain-facts/

CHAPTER 5

15 Maggie Wooll, "Don't let limiting beliefs hold you back. Learn to overcome yours", BetterUp, July 19, 2022, https://www.betterup.com/blog/what-are-limiting-beliefs

CHAPTER 6

16 Masih, Niha, "Too tired to be healthy? You're not alone, survey finds," *The Washington Post*, May 17, 2023, https://www.washington-post.com/wellness/2023/05/17/too-tired-exercise-yougov-poll/

17 Jeff Haden, *The Motivation Myth*, Portfolio/Penguin, New York, 2018.

18 Emily Guarnotta, PsyD, "What Does Dopamine Do, and How Does It Influence Behavior?," ed. India B. Gomez, PhD, goodrx.com, accessed October 25, 2021, https://www.goodrx.com/classes/dopamine-agonist/what-does-dopamine-do

CHAPTER 7

19 James Gallagher, "Fighting 40s Flab," WebMD, May 12, 2004, https://www.webmd.com/diet/features/fighting-40s-flab. James Gallagher, "Metabolism peaks at age one and tanks after 60, study finds," *BBC News*, August 12, 2021, https://www.bbc.com/news/health-58186710

20 "Introduction to Menopause," Johns Hopkins Medicine, November 19, 2019, https://www.hopkinsmedicine.org/health/conditions-and-diseases/introduction-to-menopause

21 Alexandra C. McPherron et.al., "Increasing Muscle Mass to Improve Metabolism," National Institute of Health National Library of Medicine, April 1, 2013, https://www.ncbi.nlm.nih.gov/pmc/articles/PMC3661116/

22 "Should you do cardio or lift weights?", Medical News Today, May 13, 2021, https://www.medicalnewstoday.com/articles/323922#calculating-weightlifting-calories

CHAPTER 8

23 "Prescription drugs," Georgetown University McCourt School of Public Policy Health Policy Institute, November 2023, https://hpi.georgetown.edu/rxdrugs/

24 Mayo Clinic Staff, "Triglycerides: Why do they matter?", Mayo Clinic, September 3, 2022, https://www.mayoclinic.org/diseases-conditions/high-blood-cholesterol/in-depth/triglycerides/art-20048186

25 "What is metabolic syndrome?" John Hopkins Medicine, November 2023, https://www.hopkinsmedicine.org/health/conditions-and-diseases/metabolic-syndrome

26 Andrew M Freeman, Luis A. Acevedo, Nicholas Pennings, "Insulin Resistance", National Institute of Health, National Library of Medicine, August 17, 2023, https://www.ncbi.nlm.nih.gov/books/NBK507839/

27 Mike McAvennie, "What Are Normal Testosterone Levels By Age?", The Edge Powered by Hone Health, November 22, 2023, https://honehealth.com/edge/health/testosterone-levels-by-age/

28 Valerie Paullonis,"Fact check: Testosterone levels have dropped in recent decades, but not by 50%", *USA Today*, May 9, 2022, https://www.usatoday.com/story/news/factcheck/2022/05/09/fact-check-testosterone-levels-lower-25-1999-2016/7381735001/

29 "What is Hashimoto's thyroiditis?", John Hopkins Medicine, November 2023, https://www.hopkinsmedicine.org/health/conditions-and-diseases/hashimotos-thyroiditis

30 Audrey J. Weiss, Ph.D., and Anne Elixhauser, Ph.D., "Sports-Related Emergency D/epartment Visits and Hospital Inpatient Stays, 2013", Agency for Healthcare Research and Quality, July 2016, https://hcup-us.ahrq.gov/reports/statbriefs/sb207-Sports-Hospital-Emergency-Department-2013.jsp

CHAPTER 11

31 Joey Thurman, *The Minimum Method*, BenBella Books, December 2022, Dallas, Texas.

CHAPTER 12

32 Alec McPike, "Maintaining a Healthy Weight During the Holidays: Survey", Innerbody, October 9, 2023, https://www.innerbody.com/maintaining-a-healthy-weight-during-the-holidays-survey

33 Bryan Walsh, "Why Frequent Business Travelers Are Fatter and Less Healthy", *Time*, May 3, 2011, https://healthland.time.com/2011/05/03/why-frequent-business-travelers-are-fatter-and-less-healthy/

CHAPTER 14

34 Sandy Loder, "The impact of 45,000 negative thoughts", Peak Dynamics, March 10, 2023, http://insights.peak-dynamics.net/post/102i-a4i/the-impact-of-45-000-negative-thoughts

CHAPTER 15

35 Joseph Nguyen, *Don't Believe Everything You Think*, independently published, 2022.

36 "Exercise more effective than medicines to manage mental health", University of South Australia, 24 February, 2023, https://www.unisa.edu.au/media-centre/Releases/2023/exercise-more-effective-than-medicines-to-manage-mental-health/

37 Jennifer Sokira, "Music Therapy: An Opportunity to Support Older Adults Healing from Trauma, Generations, July 19, 2023. https://generations.asaging.org/music-therapy-help-older-adults-heal-trauma

38 Charles Duhigg, *The Power of Habit*, January 2014, Random House Publishing Group, New York.

CHAPTER 16

39 Petra Kolber, *Perfection Detox*, Da Capo Lifelong Books, 2018.

CHAPTER 17

40 Dr. Michelle Segar, *No Sweat*, AMACOM, 2015.

CHAPTER 18

41 Todd M. Manini, "Energy Expenditure and Aging", National Library of Medicine, August 19, 2009, https://www.ncbi.nlm.nih.gov/pmc/articles/PMC2818133

42 Scott Frothingham, "What Is Basal Metabolic Rate?," Healthline, November 12, 2018, https://www.healthline.com/health/what-is-basal-metabolic-rate

43 Sam Milller, *Metabolism Made Simple*, Lioncrest Publishing, October 2022.

44 G. Seematter et. al., "Stress and Metabolism," https://pubmed.ncbi.nlm.nih.gov, n.d., https://pubmed.ncbi.nlm.nih.gov/18370704/

45 Sunil Sharma and Mani Kavuru, "Sleep and Metabolism: An Overview," https://www.ncbi.nlm.nih.gov, August 2 , 2010, https://www.ncbi.nlm.nih.gov/pmc/articles/PMC2929498/

46 Douglas J. Kominsky et. al., "Metabolic Shifts in Immunity and Inflammation," https://www.ncbi.nlm.nih.gov, April 15, 2010, https://www.ncbi.nlm.nih.gov/pmc/articles/PMC4077461/

47 Don Amerman, "How Does Hydration Affect Metabolism?," Healthy Eating | SF Gate, December 27, 2018, https://healthyeating.sfgate.com/hydration-affect-metabolism-2886.html

48 Tasreen Alibhai, "How Your Digestive Health Affects Your Metabolism Including Energy and Weight Loss", Vancouver Naturopath, April 30, 2017, https://vitaliahealthcare.ca/blog/digestive-health-affects-metabolism-energy-weight-loss

49 Marshall S. Runge, MD, PhD, "Weighing the Facts: The Tough Truth About Weight Loss," Michigan Medicine, University of Michigan, April 12, 2017, https://www.michiganmedicine.org/health-lab/weighing-facts-tough-truth-about-weight-loss

CHAPTER 19

50 Nazik Elgaddal, M.S., Ellen A. Kramarow, Ph.D., and Cynthia Reuben, M.A., " Physical Activity Among Adults Aged 18 and Over: United States, 2020", Centers for Disease Control and Prevention, August 2022, https://www.cdc.gov/nchs/products/databriefs/db443.htm

51 "Metabolism", The Cleveland Clinic, August 2021, https://my.clevelandclinic.org/health/body/21893-metabolism

52 Greg Nuchols, "How many additional calories does each pound of muscle burn?", Stronger by Science, June 14, 2023, https://www.strongerbyscience.com/calories-muscle-burn/

53 Jayne Leonard, "How to Build Muscle with Exercise," January 8, 2020, https://www.medicalnewstoday.com/articles/319151

54 In addition to strength training, the HIIT style of cardio can also trigger EPOC.

55 J LaForgia, R T Withers, C J Gore, "Efffects of exercise intensity and duration on the excess post-exercise oxygen consumption", National Library of Medicine, December 24, 2006, https://pubmed.ncbi.nlm.nih.gov/17101527/

56 "What Is EPOC?," Larson Sports and Orthopaedics, May 4, 2018, https://larsonsportsortho.com/what-is-epoc/

57 Jeremy Ethier, "Should You Be Training To Failure? (AVOID THIS MISTAKE!)", June 7, 2020, https://builtwithscience.com/fitness-tips/training-to-failure/

58 Andre Adams, "Progressive Overload Explained: Grow Muscle & Strength Today," National Academy of Sports Medicine (NASM), 2022, https://blog.nasm.org/progressive-overload-explained

CHAPTER 20

59 Beth Mole, "90% of US has a poor diet, and 25% doesn't exercise", Ars Technica, January 24, 2022, https://arstechnica.com/science/2022/01/even-before-covid-americans-were-failing-at-health-basics-diet-exercise/

60 This title is mostly tongue-in-cheek. Please do not take this to mean that you can never have these things, or that if you have them you are sinning. It's merely meant to give you an easy way to remember the foods to limit.

CHAPTER 21

61 "Sleep by the Numbers," National Sleep Foundation, May 12, 2021, https://www.thensf.org/sleep-facts-and-statistics/

62 Matthew Walker, PhD, *Why We Sleep: Unlocking the Power of Sleep and Dreams*, October 2017, Scribner.

63 Dr. Teofilo Lee-Chiong, M.D., Dr. Mark Aloia, Ph.D., Dr. David White, M.D., "Globla Sleep Survey: The global pursuit of better sleep health", Philips, 2019, https://www.usa.philips.com/c-dam/b2c/master/experience/smartsleep/world-sleep-day/2019/2019-philips-world-sleep-day-survey-results.pdf

64 "Energy Efficient Scheduling for Mobile Push Notifications", ResearchGate, August 2015, https://www.researchgate.net/figure/Number-of-Notifications-per-User-per-Day_fig2_299931683

65 "Can't Shed Those Pounds?", WebMD, 2023, https://www.webmd.com/obesity/features/sleep-weight-loss

66 WebMD Editorial Contributors, "What Happens to Your Body When You Sleep?", WebMD, March 13, 2021, https://www.webmd.com/sleep-disorders/what-happens-body-during-sleep

67 Danielle Pacheco, Dr. Abhinav Singh, "Exercise and Sleep", SleepFoundation.org, October 11, 2023, https://www.sleepfoundation.org/physical-activity/exercise-and-sleep

CHAPTER 23

68 Scott Hensley, "Poll: Americans Say We're Angrier Than A Generation Ago", *NPR*, June 26, 2019, https://www.npr.org/sections/health-shots/2019/06/26/735757156/poll-americans-say-were-angrier-than-a-generation-ago

69 "Always Connected: How Smartphones And Social Keep Us Engaged," IDC Research Report Sponsored By Facebook, Doc. #24043, 2013.

70 Hilary Achauer, "Why Are We All Still Watching TV Right Before Bed?", SleepFoundation.org, July 8, 2022, https://www.sleepfoundation.org/sleep-news/watching-tv-before-sleep-most-popular-bedtime-routine

CHAPTER 24

71 "Americans reveal what they would do with more free time: poll", *New York Post*, January 24, 2023, https://nypost.com/2023/01/24/americans-reveal-what-they-would-do-with-more-free-time-poll/

CHAPTER 26

72 Robert Kiyosaki, *Rich Dad, Poor Dad,* Plata Publishing, 2017.

www.ingramcontent.com/pod-product-compliance
Lightning Source LLC
Chambersburg PA
CBHW050449270326
41927CB00009B/1662
* 9 7 9 8 9 8 9 3 1 4 9 1 1 *